Rapid Recovery
from Back and Neck Pain

A Nine-Step Recovery Plan

Rapid Recovery from Back and Neck Pain

A Nine-Step Recovery Plan

FRED AMIR, R.E.H.S.

Health Advisory Group, LLC
Santa Clara, California

Published by
Health Advisory Group, LLC
2464 El Camino Real, PMB 157
Santa Clara, CA 95051
www.rapidrecovery.net

Library of Congress Catalog Card Number
98-094189

ISBN Number
0-9669826-0-6

ABOUT THE AUTHOR

Fred Amir is the recipient of the University of California's Knowles Ryerson Award for Leadership, a registered environmental health specialist, and the founder and president of *Health Solutions*.

Health Solutions is a health consulting and educational firm specializing in empowering individuals with knowledge and strategies to maximize their innate abilities for better health. Fred's seminars, titled *Rapid Recovery from Chronic Pain, The Road to Wellness,* and *Living by Design,* have helped others recover rapidly to live pain-free and much healthier and happier lives. He has conducted seminars for the University of California, CIGNA Group Insurance, Iowa State University, and other organizations.

Fred is an avid reader who believes in life-long learning and is a student of martial arts, having studied kenpo karate and tae kwon do. He lives with his wife and two children in the greater San Jose area.

CONTENTS

ACKNOWLEDGMENTS

My deep gratitude and thanks to Dr. John E. Sarno, Professor of Clinical Rehabilitation Medicine at New York University, for taking the time to review my manuscript and for his valuable comments. I am also enormously indebted to Lee Esquibel, Director of Santa Clara County Department of Environmental Health, for reviewing the manuscript, despite his busy schedule, and for his counsel and support. My thanks to Leode Franklin, Director of Santa Clara County Environmental Resources Agency, as well for her support and advice for improving the text.

I would also like to extend a special thanks to Judy McConnell of the University of California, Office of The President; Joseph Capizzi of CIGNA Group Insurance; Dr. Fred Rahbar of Iowa State University; Barbara Fain of the Santa Clara County Wellness Program; Dr. Amr Mohsen of Aptix Corporation; and Dr. Hamdi El-Sissi of Phylon Communications, for their support and encouragement.

I am very grateful to Anthony Dymond, Ph.D., and Lura Dymond, not only for their insightful comments, but also for many years of friendship and encouragement. As an editor, Ms. Dymond has been an invaluable source of advice and guidance throughout this work. I would like to add my special thanks to Judith Moretz and Cathy Cambron for their editorial skills. I am also grateful for the comments and encouragement I received from Jere Conley and appreciate the helpful suggestions given by Walter Kleine.

My love and gratitude to my wife, Farah, for her patience throughout this work and for watching the children while I spent many nights and weekends at the computer, not to mention the many hours she spent proofreading.

Also, many thanks to my dear friend, Jamaal Zarabozo, who typed the initial draft of the manuscript, and, interestingly enough, recovered from back pain in the process! Incidentally, Judy Moretz and Cathy Cambron also recovered from back pain and shoulder pain, respectively, while editing the manuscript! I wish them all the best of faith, health, wealth, and happiness.

INTRODUCTION

*R*apid recovery from back and neck pain?! Sounds too good to be possible. But it is. I know, because I have experienced this phenomenon firsthand. After months of suffering from chronic pain in my back, neck, legs, knees, arms, and hands, and total disability—after months of going from one doctor to another with no cure in sight—I was able to recover within four days to live an active and productive life. Others with recurrent or chronic pain have also experienced this rapid recovery following the proven techniques described in this book.

This book provides you with the scientific research on the cause of most back, neck, and hand pain and shows how you can get rid of the pain quickly and easily. Those who have attended my seminars on rapid recovery from chronic pain and have applied these techniques have noticed significant improvements within a few hours to a few days, and complete recovery shortly afterward.

Skeptical? A healthy dose of skepticism is a good thing. I am very scientific-minded and skeptical myself. When I'm presented with new ideas and new possibilities, though, I do my best to keep an open mind—especially when it comes to my health. I ask you to do the same. Question what you read, but be open to new possibilities. The only way you are ever going to get well is to take charge of this debilitating condition, by learning all you can about it and being willing to take action. Indeed, knowledge is power!

If you suffer from chronic or recurrent back, neck, or hand pain, you know how difficult it can be to find a cure. If you are frustrated, as I was, by the ineffective treatments you have received and want to live a pain-free life again, this book will show you how. It takes you along on my search, like a detective's, for clues to solve the mystery of my back pain—a mystery because back pain baffles even doctors and surgeons who specialize in treating it. The frustrated patients of these back pain specialists, instead of getting answers or effective treatment, may hear: "Well, that's how back pain is!" Or worse: "You just have to learn to live with it."

In contrast, this book will tell you about the revolutionary discovery and treatment program from New York University and give you a nine-step rapid recovery plan made up of easy yet highly effective techniques used by Olympic athletes.

HOW YOU WILL BENEFIT

How can the concepts and techniques presented in this book help you? To put it simply, if you follow the rapid recovery plan presented here, you can expect to benefit in the following ways:

- You can become pain-free, as you learn how to eliminate chronic pain quickly and easily.
- You can become more active and productive, as you live free of the limitations brought on by chronic pain.
- You can become much healthier, because following this plan leads to many other improvements in your health as well.
- You will be much happier, not just as you become healthier, but also as you learn many new skills that can make a tremendous difference in all aspects of your life.

Most of these benefits emerge within a few days—even within a few hours—if you follow the concepts and techniques explained here. These techniques are so effective that you may notice improvements in your level of mobility and pain even before you finish this book. I have seen this phenomenon in those with whom I have had the privilege of sharing this information.

You might be asking yourself, "How can people who have suffered months and years of chronic pain, who have probably tried all kinds of treatments with little success, recover so quickly?" I will answer this question in some detail in the next few pages and in depth in this book. I understand if you are skeptical. But keep an open mind; read and evaluate what you read carefully. I will provide you the scientific research and proven techniques every step of the way.

Also, keep in mind that I have been there: in pain, night and day—pain in my back, neck, legs, knees, arms, and hands. I was so disabled that I could not climb three steps or write two lines, and I wondered whether I would ever be free of pain again. But I recovered rapidly and completely and now help others by teaching these techniques in my seminars and workshops.

Besides my own recovery, over and over again I have seen men and women who had been told that their conditions were permanent, or that they had to have surgery, improve overnight and recover within a few days following these techniques. Among them is a forty-year-old who is a Stanford graduate in electrical engineering and a professor at the University of California. He suffered from neck pain and numbness in his right arm and fingers. The neurosurgeon had recommended neck surgery for a bulging disc, based on the MRI findings. But once the professor learned the concepts and techniques presented in this book, he recovered quickly and avoided surgery.

And then there was the facility manager who was diagnosed with carpal tunnel syndrome in both hands. Surgery on his right wrist had done little to improve his condition. Following only two of the steps in the nine-step recovery plan helped him improve overnight and recover within a few days. He cancelled the surgery for his left wrist and has been free of pain for more than three years. There are many others, and you can read the letters they sent me in Appendix B.

BACK FACTS KEPT SECRET!

If you have read the back-pain literature, you have probably come across the following facts:

- Eight out of ten adults suffer from back pain at some point in their lives.
- Back problems are second only to sore throat as this nation's most common ailment.
- Nineteen million doctor visits are made for back pain annually.
- Eight million new cases of back pain occur every year.
- Back pain is the leading cause of work-related disability.

As I searched the medical literature for information on back pain, however, I discovered some very amazing statistics—statistics rarely found in books on back pain and usually not mentioned by back specialists. Did you know the following surprising facts?

- "Surgery has been found to be helpful in only 1 in 100 cases of low back pain. In some people, surgery can even cause more problems." So concluded the Agency for Health Care Policy and Research of the U.S. Department of Health and Human Services after conducting a comprehensive study of more than 10,000 cases of back pain.[1] Even though I knew back surgery was not a very effective treatment for most people, I was a little shocked to learn that 99 percent of the time it fails to help patients.
- "Injecting methylyprednisolone acetate [cortisone] into the facet joints is of little value in the treatment of patients with chronic low back pain." This was the conclusion of a study published in *The New England Journal of Medi-*

---

[1] U.S. Department of Health and Human Services, Agency for Health Care Policy and Research, *Understanding Acute Low Back Pain Problems,* Publication No. 95-0644 (Rockville, Md.: December 1994), p. 12.

cine.[2] Researchers found no significant improvement in patients who received a cortisone shot compared to those who were given a shot of saline solution (salt water) in their facet joints or herniated discs![3]

- "Treatments [for whiplash-associated disorders] evaluated in a rigorous manner show little or no evidence of efficacy." This finding was the result of an exhaustive study conducted at McGill University.[4] Researchers found treatments ranging from neck collar to traction to be of little or no value.[5]

Even though these surprising facts have appeared in some of the most authoritative and prestigious medical journals, you will not learn this crucial information from most back and neck specialists, inside or outside the medical profession. Indeed, these treatments are used so widely that you may be shocked to learn that they don't work! So take a minute to read over these conclusions of respected medical experts again, to empower yourself to make better decisions regarding your treatment options and avoid ineffective surgeries and shots.[6]

---

[2] Caretter, S., et al., "A Controlled Trial of Corticosteriod Injections into Facet Joints for Chronic Low Vack Pain," *The New England Journal of Medicine* 325 (1991): 1001–1007.

[3] Another such study titled, "Epidural Corticosteriod Injections for Sciatica due to Herniated Nucleus Pulposus," *The New England Journal of Medicine* 336 (1997):1634–1640, concluded that cortisone injections to relieve sciatica caused by a herniated disc "offer no significant functional benefit" compared to saline solution injections.

[4] Spitzer, W.O., et al., "Scientific Monograph of the Quebec Task Force on Whiplash-Associated Disorders," *Spine* 20 (1995): 34S-39S.

[5] Surgery for carpal tunnel syndrome has also been found ineffective: "Correcting carpal tunnel syndrome is one of the most common operations performed today. The only problem is, it often doesn't work," concluded researchers at the Washington University School of Medicine in St. Louis ("Surgery Often Useless for Carpal Tunnel Pain," *San Jose Mercury News*, February 22, 1995.)

[6] A machinist who attended one of my seminars told me that his surgeon had quoted him an 80 percent success rate for back surgery. The

Why is it that conventional treatments fail to cure back and neck pain? Because, as *The New England Journal of Medicine* puts it, "Up to 85 percent of patients with low back pain cannot be given a definitive diagnosis."[7] That's right—up to 85 percent! No wonder most of these treatments fail. As the saying goes, "Correct diagnosis is half the cure!" Without the right diagnosis, how can we expect an effective treatment? As you will see in this section, according to the published scientific research most of the common diagnoses for chronic back pain are unfounded.

You can already see that this book is unique in its approach to back pain. The crucial valuable information set out here results from years of research into the causes and treatments for back, neck, and hand pain. This is information that you can use immediately and benefit from for the rest of your life. At the very least, because of what you have learned so far, you can avoid useless, faddish treatments that actually may do more harm than good.

The possibility that treatments for back pain may actually create additional problems was addressed in a revealing article, "Fads in the Treatment of Low Back Pain," published in the prestigious *The New England Journal of Medicine.* Dr. Richard Deyo wrote: "Recent clinical trials have challenged the efficacy of many popular treatments, including bed rest, traction, and transcutaneous electrical nerve stimulation. Such fads are not in-

---

machinist was furious when he learned that back surgery is helpful only 1 percent of the time and can actually cause more problems than it resolves. He avoided surgery and recovered rapidly when he began following the nine-step rapid recovery plan. You might know someone whose condition improved or who possibly recovered as a result of surgery or a cortisone shot. Remember, the findings discussed here were drawn from large-scale studies and group comparisons of patients. You might ask yourself, "Why is it that one treatment for the same diagnosis works for some and not for others?" This is, of course, one of those mysteries of back pain that this book will explain in detail.

[7] Jensen, M.C., et al., "Magnetic Resonance Imaging of the Lumbar Spine in People Without Back Pain," *The New England Journal of Medicine* 331 (1994): 69–73.

nocuous; they may lead to unnecessary morbidity and costs, as well as to embarrassment for professionals."[8]

But my aim in this book is not simply to help you avoid useless treatments. In addition, the book provides you with empowering concepts and effective techniques for a rapid and complete recovery. Just imagine being free of pain: moving freely without pain as your guide; sitting and sleeping comfortably; feeling young and healthy again. These are some of the many wonderful benefits I have enjoyed since my rapid recovery, and I believe you will too.

CORRECT DIAGNOSIS IS HALF THE CURE!

I already mentioned how crucial a correct diagnosis is for treatment of recurrent and chronic back pain. Before we go any further, I would like to share with you a bit of medical history.

Back pain has become a very frustrating health problem for individuals as well as for the society at large. However, the history of medicine contains other examples of devastating problems with simple solutions. For example: Imagine it is nineteenth-century France. The country is facing a serious public health problem. Women are dying of childbirth fever. So many are dying that one hospital has to be closed for a month while doctors try to discover the cause. Finally one man, a chemist by training, makes the correct diagnosis and prescribes a very effective treatment. This man is Louis Pasteur.

Pasteur determines that the cause of childbirth fever and death is pathogens (germs) spread by doctors and nurses from one patient to another. He offers a very simple and effective solution: doctors and nurses must wash their hands prior to delivering each baby and between patients. He is ridiculed and ignored. Experts of the time taunt Pasteur: "How can tiny germs we cannot see

---

[8] Deyo, R., "Fads in the Treatment of Low Back Pain," *The New England Journal of Medicine* 325 (1991): 1039-1040.

with our naked eyes actually cause disease and death?" "How can the simple act of washing our hands make a difference?"

The "experts" of Pasteur's day could understand how tiny insects can sting or bite and harm people, but they were not willing to open their minds to the possibility that smaller organisms can also cause harm and disease. Only God knows how many women died in childbirth until Pasteur's solution was put in practice and handwashing became standard procedure in all hospitals. Millions of lives are saved every year because of Pasteur's discovery.

In this example, as in the case of back pain, correct diagnosis of a devastating problem can lead to an almost unbelievably simple, very effective solution. Lack of a correct diagnosis is the number-one reason back pain has become such a serious health problem. As mentioned earlier, as many as 85 percent of patients with low back pain never receive a definitive diagnosis. Without a definitive diagnosis, a cure cannot be expected; however, once we have the correct diagnosis, the solution is simple! This is the reason that people who have learned the diagnosis and the simple, effective recovery techniques presented in this book have been able to recover so rapidly from months and years of chronic pain.

As I mentioned earlier, everything I explain here is backed by solid scientific research, but for you to get the most benefit from this book, I ask you to keep an open mind and be willing to consider new possibilities when it comes to understanding the cause and treatment of chronic back, neck, and hand pain. I want you to be one of those people who are pioneers in recognizing new life-enhancing discoveries and who are among the first to embrace them. Having said that, I think you will nevertheless find this book takes a fundamentally common sense approach to diagnosing and treating back and neck pain.

Now let me tell you a little bit about myself: how I began my search for answers, learned how to recover rapidly, and resumed a pain-free, active life.

MY BAD BACK

As one who suffered from chronic back pain, I am all too familiar with the agony and disability it brings. In addition to living through more than two years of back pain, I developed pain in my neck, both legs, knees, elbows, and one shoulder; suffered gastritis due to my use of prescription and over-the-counter anti-inflammatory medications; and experienced other health problems as well.

I was seen by general practitioners as well as back specialists and even a nationally known orthopedic surgeon. Each one had his own diagnosis. I was diagnosed with osteoarthritis of the spine, degenerated discs, sprained back muscles, pinched nerve, herniated disc, leaky discs, and piriformis syndrome as possible causes for my back and leg pain. I was given a wide variety of different medications and treatments, some of which made my condition worse.[9]

I was constantly in pain and became severely disabled. At one point the pain was so severe that I was not able to stand or sit for more that fifteen minutes at a time, to climb three steps, to walk farther than one hundred yards, to carry more than four pounds, to lift a half-gallon milk container, or even to write two lines. My life became limited in ways that I had never imagined. I had to stay away from work and was faced with serious questions about my career, my future, and my life, especially as a husband and father.

---

[9] I was too skeptical to try nonconventional treatments such as chiropractic, acupuncture, or other alternative treatments. Although I met people who found these treatments helpful, none of them were permanently cured and all required further treatments, sometimes several times a week. So both conventional medical and alternative treatments appeared ineffective to me.

SEARCH FOR ANSWERS

Early in this painful and often frustrating ordeal I discovered that the medical professionals themselves were baffled by back pain. Not only did they have difficulty making a proper diagnosis and prescribing effective treatment, but they were not even capable of providing satisfactory answers to my simplest questions about back pain:

- Why are the majority of people with back pain or chronic pain under fifty years old?
- Why, unlike a broken bone, does back pain not heal, instead often lasting for years?
- If weak muscles are the cause, how strong do back muscles have to be for one to recover? Do we all need to become bodybuilders to be free of pain?
- If improper sitting and bending can damage the back, why aren't gymnasts and other athletes who put tremendous pressure on their spines all suffering from debilitating back pain?

To these and many other questions, which appeared simple enough for back specialists and experts to resolve, the responses were unconvincing answers, shrugged shoulders, or simply: "Well, that's how back pain is!"

In the face of the medical community's apparent ineptitude in treating back pain—and the fact that some of the treatments prescribed for me actually made my condition worse—I realized that I could no longer afford to be a passive patient. I began to take an active role in my diagnosis and treatment, and tried to become an informed consumer, searching the available literature for a cure to my disabling condition—a condition so prevalent that it has become a national health problem.

Most books and articles on back pain echoed what I was told by my doctors and therapists. Most of what I read attributed the pain to some spinal disorder or to weak muscles, and advised the use of proper body mechanics, good posture, and exercise as means to prevent and improve back problems. Some authors mentioned proper diet, acupressure, meditation, and reducing stress as helpful. Although the information I found helped me avoid unnecessary tests and treatments, I was not able to find answers to my questions about back pain—let alone a cure. At times it seemed I would have to live with pain and disability for years, if not the rest of my life.

AN ANSWER—AT LAST!

Finally, after months of searching and reading I learned about Dr. John Sarno's discovery at New York University. Dr. Sarno, a professor of clinical rehabilitation medicine at the New York University School of Medicine, has treated thousands of back patients for more than twenty years. Prior to his discovery, Dr. Sarno had been puzzled by back pain for many years. He was troubled by the fact that treatments often failed to cure the patient.

He noticed that the pain and physical examination findings often did not correlate. For example, a patient with a lumbar disc that was herniated to the left might exhibit right-leg pain; or a disc pressed on a nerve energizing the foot muscles, but the pain or numbness was felt in the back of the leg and buttocks as well! So Dr. Sarno concluded that more was involved than simply one disc pressing on a particular nerve. I will discuss in detail later the physiological changes that cause pain and numbness in the back, neck, and hands, and how the pain becomes chronic.

As he looked deeper into the medical histories of his patients, Dr. Sarno discovered something that is often neglected by most medical professionals. He noticed that 88 percent of his patients had histories of disorders such as migraine headaches, colitis, stomach ulcers, hay fever, asthma, eczema, and high blood pressure. These disorders were strongly suspected of being caused by chronic repressed anger, anxiety, worries, frustrations, stress, and tension. Dr. Sarno wondered whether, in the same way that chronic anger, anxiety, worries, and frustrations can cause physiological changes leading to these physical symptoms, back pain could also be a physical manifestation of such negative emotions. So he put this new diagnosis to work and began treating his patients accordingly. Of course, at first the majority of his patients felt there was not enough stress and tension in their lives to cause their pain. Many of them also felt they were handling their teenage children, problems at work, and marital problems effectively. However, as Dr. Sarno talked to them more they developed a better awareness of how those same bothersome issues were actually creating a great deal of negative feelings deep inside, and how these feelings were causing physiological changes that caused the pain—real, debilitating pain.[10]

Once Dr. Sarno treated back patients for this new diagnosis and not for some structural abnormality, his patients began to recover. Of his patients with confirmed cases of herniated discs, 88 percent recovered completely, while another 10 percent improved significantly—without surgery. Thus, Dr. Sarno's patients with confirmed cases of herniated discs experienced a recovery rate of almost 98 percent—certainly a much better result than the 1 percent success rate experienced with surgery.[11]

---

[10] The renowned author and physician Dr. Andrew Weil is a great proponent of Dr. Sarno's diagnosis. In fact, he has devoted an entire chapter in his book *Spontaneous Healing* to explaining the diagnosis. As he put it in his newsletter *Self Healing,* "Sarno makes a strong case that most back pain is the result of the mind's interference with normal functioning of the nerves and blood circulation to muscles, a condition called Tension Myositis Syndrome, or TMS. . . . I am a great believer in TMS, having seen many cases of chronic back pain disappear as if by magic with major life changes such as a new romance or a new job. . . . In my opinion, all chronic back (and neck) pain should be considered TMS until proven otherwise" (October 1997, pp. 1–3).

[11] An important study published in *The New England Journal of Medicine* and reported by the *New York Times* (Jensen, M.C., et al.,"Magnetic Resonance Imaging of the Lumbar Spine in People Without Back Pain," *The New England Journal of Medicine* 331 (1994): 69–73) raised serious doubts about herniated disc or other spinal abnormalities being responsible for back pain; the researchers used magnetic resonance imaging to examine the spines of 98 men and women who had no back pain. They found that nearly two-thirds of

NOT ME!

I know what most of you are thinking: "Not me!" That was exactly my response to the notion that tension and stress were causing my pain. Being a calm, positive person who rarely gets angry or tense, I was quite skeptical about whether Dr. Sarno's findings applied to me. It is well known that stress and tension can aggravate back pain and many other disorders. However, could repressed anger, anxiety, worries, and frustrations be the actual cause of so much pain and disability? I figured I had nothing to lose by keeping an open mind and learning more. At the very least maybe what I learned could help someone else. As I learned more about Dr. Sarno's explanation of the pattern of pain,

---

the subjects had spinal abnormalities, including bulging or protruding disks, herniated discs, degenerated discs, spondylolysis, and stenosis of the central canal. The prevalence of bulges and protrusions was highest at the L4-5 and L5-S1 vertebrae of the lumbar spine. This study raised serious doubts about the commonly used methods of diagnosing and treating back pain and concluded that there seems to be no correlation between back abnormalities and back pain.

Moreover, this was not the first study to reveal that there is no correlation between the existence of a spinal abnormality and back pain. The following is a list of other studies conducted over the last four decades that demonstrate this fact: McRae, D. L., "Asymptomatic Intervertebral Disc Protrusions," *acta radiol* 46 (1956): 9–27; Hitselberger, W. E., et al., "Abnormal Myelograms in Asymptomatic Patients," *Journal of Neurosurgery* 28 (1968): 204–206; Wiesel, S. W., et al., "The Incidence of Positive CAT Scans in an Asymptomatic Group of Patients," *Spine* 9 (1984): 549–551; Powel, M. C., et al., "Prevalence of Lumbar Disc Degeneration Observed by Magnetic Resonance in Symptomless Women," *Lancet* 2 (1986): 1366–1377; Weinred, J. C., et al., "Prevalence of Lumbosacral Intervertebral Disk Abnormalities on MR Images in Pregnant and Asymptomatic Nonpregnant Women," *Radiology* 170 (1989): 125–128; Boden, S. D., et al., "Abnormal Magnetic Resonance Scans of the Lumbar Spine in Asymptomatic Subjects," *Journal of Bone Joint Surgery* 72 (1990): 403–408.

how it becomes chronic, and my other concerns, I found convincing answers to all my questions and more.[12]

I began to see why so many people under the age of fifty facing career and family responsibilities suffer from chronic pain; why, unlike a broken bone that heals, back pain becomes chronic and can last for years; why we do not see an epidemic of disabling back and leg pain among Olympic and professional athletes who put tremendous pressure on their spines; and why, because the mind/body connection is so often neglected, the causes of as much as 85 percent of back pain are not clear. Dr. Sarno's explanation, of course, makes it clear why surgery and most treatments directed at correcting "spinal abnormalities" fail.

It was indeed a relief for me to learn that our spines are not so fragile, and that we do not have to spend the rest of our lives worrying about our posture and how we sit and move so as not to hurt our backs again. Interestingly enough, a recent study of four thousand postal workers compared those who had attended back schools with those who received no such training.[13] The study found that such training did not reduce the rate of low back injury, cost per injury, time off from work per injury, rate of related injuries, or rate of repeated injury after return to work. Researchers concluded that there were "no long-term benefits associated with training."[14]

---

[12] We all are well aware how severe stress affects our bodies. We all have experienced butterflies in our stomachs before a presentation or a job interview. We all have felt the rapid heartbeat or sweaty hands when stopped for speeding. In such situations we can clearly see the connection between changes in our emotions and changes in our bodies. However, when experiencing low-level chronic anger, anxiety, and stress, the physical symptoms are much more subtle and may not manifest themselves until much later, sometimes at night or the following day.

[13] Back schools are educational programs developed by physical therapists for patients with back pain; these schools teach good posture for sitting and standing, and stretching and strengthening exercises.

[14] Daltroy, Lawren H., et al., "A Controlled Trial of an Educational

Now we can add training for good posture and back exercises to the long list of unproven and ineffective approaches to treating and preventing back pain. Isn't it great that we don't have to worry about our posture or do those boring back stretches for the rest of our lives?

The freedom that comes with this knowledge is wonderful. Certainly we must use good judgment and proper lifting techniques to prevent back injury, for like any other part of our body our backs can be injured. But in the same way that other parts of our body heal after an injury, so do our backs. Here we are concerned about back pain that does not end for months and years regardless of the initial cause, whether it was a car accident, lifting something heavy or light, or just "sleeping wrong"—waking up in pain one morning.

Back pain is a very common human response to repressed anger, anxiety, frustration, and tension. This explains why millions suffer from it, and why those in the prime of their lives, faced with the tensions and anxieties of raising a family and with job responsibilities, are more prone to back pain than people in other age groups. Nevertheless, back pain is a problem that can afflict any age group.

KIDS GET IT TOO!

Whereas eight out of ten adults suffer from back pain at some point in their lives, nearly 36 percent of American adolescents suffer from low back pain by the age of fifteen, according to a study published in the *American Journal of Public Health*.[15] This large number should not come as a surprise. Just consider the amount of peer pressure, stress, and anxiety teenagers face in today's society, and it becomes clear why they too suffer from

---

Program to Prevent Low Back Injuries," *The New England Journal of Medicine* 337 (1997): 332–338.

[15] Olsen, Todd L., et al., "The Epidemiology of Low Back Pain in an Adolescent Population," *American Journal of Public Health* 82 (April 1992): 606–608.

back pain. In contrast, it is hard to believe that degenerative spinal problems could possibly be responsible for such a significant percentage of teenagers experiencing back pain.

RAPID RECOVERY

Dr. Sarno provided clear, convincing answers to my questions about back pain and its recurrence and chronicity. His studies solved the back pain puzzle for me. However, his treatment program takes about two to six weeks to take effect. For reasons I will explain in the book, I did not want to wait that long. I also felt, based on my studies in psychology and achievement, that the treatment program could be greatly enhanced by incorporating techniques used by Olympic athletes.

Therefore, I combined his treatment program with my knowledge of psychology and many years of personal experience with the workings of the mind to design an effective nine-step rapid recovery plan. This plan enabled me to begin my journey toward a pain-free and able life immediately. Employing techniques used by Olympic athletes and high achievers, I began to reverse the physiological changes that caused the pain and made it chronic.

My improvements could be seen daily and astonished those who knew how disabled I had been before. Within the first four days of my recovery I was able to stand, bend, sit, and sleep comfortably. I was also able to walk without a limp, climb stairs, wear a tie, exercise on a cross-country ski machine, and swim. The climax of my recovery was when, less than two weeks later, I was able to carry both my children, each weighing over forty pounds. This I had not been able to do for over two years due to pain in my back, legs, knees, and arms. It felt wonderful. And one month later I began taking karate lessons.

But there was more. I had suffered from hay fever for seventeen years and had taken antihistamines to control my sneezing and itchy, watery eyes. However, with my new understanding that hay fever is one of the many disorders caused by tension, using the strategies in my nine-step recovery plan I was able to eliminate it quickly.

Then, during a routine eye exam the ophthalmologist told me that my eyes were fine, and I no longer needed the reading glasses I had been wearing for the past fourteen years! I was so surprised that I sought a second opinion. The second ophthalmologist confirmed the diagnosis. Here too I discovered that tension played a key role. In fact, decades ago, noted ophthalmologist Dr. William Bates recognized the relationship between tension and nearsightedness and other changes in the eye refraction. He designed a program for reversing the effects of tension on the eyes and eliminating the need for glasses.

Needless to say, at times I was amazed and overwhelmed by these improvements in my health in such a short time. Others have also experienced such improvements in their health. So can you! What is so wonderful about the information presented in this book is that it can help you not only to recover rapidly from chronic pain, but to enjoy many other significant improvements in your health as well. Just as the simple act of handwashing can prevent the transmission of so many diseases caused by micro-organisms, the techniques presented in this book can help you prevent as well as reverse the many physical effects of stress and tension.

WHAT YOU WILL LEARN

In the pages that follow, you will learn:
1. Why simply bending to pick up a pen can bring on back pain
2. The physiological change that causes most chronic back, neck, and hand pain
3. Why you hurt when you hurt and how the pain becomes chronic
4. Why people respond differently to various treatments
5. The treatment program from New York University
6. Related research on mind/body medicine from Harvard, Stanford, UCLA, and other major universities

7. The techniques in the nine-step rapid recovery plan, and how the techniques used by Olympic athletes can help you eliminate pain quickly and easily

8. How you can design your personal rapid recovery plan, with an entire section devoted to guiding you step-by-step through the plan

9. The mind/body connection and how to utilize it for better health

10. How you can prevent recurrence of pain by learning and applying easy and effective techniques to resolve conflicts and handle people and situations that are sources of chronic anger, frustrations, stress, and tension

11. Simple yet powerful one-minute techniques that help you deal effectively with daily sources of stress and tension for a much healthier and happier life

These concepts and techniques can accelerate the recovery process by days or weeks for most back patients. In my case these techniques brought about immediate improvements. You will see that others who have applied them have also experienced rapid improvements, in some cases overnight. Still others were able to avoid surgery and recover.

I have to admit I was also quite surprised at how easily I could resolve the same issues that were sources of chronic anger and anxiety in my life in order to live much more happily and healthily. I will also share those empowering concepts with you so that you too can enjoy better health and greater happiness.

WHAT YOU CAN EXPECT

The first two chapters of this book give a brief history of how my back pain began and how, due to improper diagnosis and treatment, I became almost completely disabled. I tell about my experiences with different doctors, therapists, and back specialists. I also share the valuable lessons I learned as a patient and a consumer so that you will not have to suffer the same difficulties that my family and I endured for so many months. The third chapter deals with my introduction and initial reaction to the concept of repressed anger, anxiety, frustration, and tension as the cause of most back pain, my further research into this concept's validity, and how my findings provided convincing answers to my questions.

Then in Chapter Four I describe my rapid recovery plan. This chapter also contains a journal in which I recount how my plan translated into daily noticeable improvements, and demonstrates how the plan may serve as a model for others who want to recover from chronic back pain.

I have dedicated the fifth chapter to the sources of tension in my life, which were the real cause of my pain. These were nothing uncommon, as we all experience problems and tensions in our relationships with our parents, spouses, children, friends, and co-workers. What is important is to realize our limitations in our capacities to please others and to cope with chronic stress.

It is also vital to understand that as calm and in control as we might appear on a conscious level, there is a part of us all deep within, on the subconscious level, that may resent certain aspects of a relationship or a situation, be it at home or work. Unless those bothersome issues are resolved through mutual respect and good communication, or through positive changes in our circumstances, it is quite natural to expect physical manifestations of the repressed anger, anxiety, and tension in the form of bodily aches and pains.

This chapter will elucidate the connection between emotions and health. Fortunately, this connection has received more attention in recent years. Medical researchers at Harvard, Stanford, Duke, and other major universities have been conducting research with fascinating results, demonstrating not only how chronic exposure to stressful circumstances can lead to health problems, but also how positive emotions such as joy, love, and hope, and having faith and communicating well with others, can help prevent disease as well as facilitate recovery. Indeed, it has been shown that we are far more in control of the workings of our bodies than previously suspected. Bill Moyers' book and public television series, *Healing and the Mind,* was another milestone along the road to a better public understanding of this concept.

It should be pointed out that undoubtedly some pain is actually caused by genuine physical disorders and injuries. It is imperative to consult proper medical professionals in order to rule out tumors, infection, bone disease, or another physical problem as the cause of pain.

Chapter Six presents the nine-step rapid recovery plan, as well as cases of men and women who have recovered rapidly by following the plan. They include:

- A Stanford graduate and University of California professor with neck pain and numbness in his right arm and fingers was diagnosed with a bulging disc
- The owner of an electrical equipment company who had a herniated disc and suffered from back and leg pain for three years
- A dentist with ten years of upper back pain and one year of leg pain
- A young businessman who suffered from eleven years of back and leg pain following two car accidents
- A manager with carpal tunnel syndrome in both hands
- A test engineer who suffered whiplash in a car accident
- A president of a computer company who suffered from three years of foot pain
- An obstetrician/gynecologist who suffered from knee pain

As you shall see, these nine steps are easy, safe, quite effective, and take little time to do. The purpose and benefits of each step are explained, and helpful action items are provided. In addition, at the end of Chapter Six you will find a daily action plan, which incorporates the nine steps in a simple and easy-to-follow format. These strategies, action items, and the daily plan will give you the tools to facilitate your start on the recovery plan, as they have done for many others. I have also provided the additional material for personalizing your recovery plan in Appendix A.

I believe the nine-step plan can help anyone who is truly motivated to rid himself or herself of pain. Unfortunately, nowadays we have come to expect a magic pill for every health problem, and we live with a medical system that rarely encourages active participation by the patient. The belief that we play an important role in our own treatment can help us make a difference, and those who are truly motivated and willing to take the necessary steps toward better health can expect a quick recovery.

These planning tools, combined with the recovery journal in Chapter Four, will give you a complete understanding of the nine steps and how they can work for you. These can also be applied to recover from other tension-related symptoms. In addition to recovery from their back pain, the people discussed in this book have also been able to reduce or eliminate other tension-related symptoms such as hay fever, canker sores, headaches, and teeth grinding during sleep. They have also noticed improvements in their immune systems, as they caught fewer colds.

I have also had the privilege of helping in the rapid recovery of a college professor who suffered from seven years of chronic bronchitis and coughed constantly, and a design manager with hereditary hemorrhagic telangiectasia (a hereditary disease characterized by profuse bleeding from nose or other areas) triggered by tension.

Since most back pain is caused by tension, I searched for strategies and methods to reduce and eliminate it. In Chapter Seven you will find nine steps for establishing good communication and resolving conflicts with your loved ones as well as others, eleven strategies for coping with stress and tension, four steps for immediately improving a marriage, and a three-step plan for raising well-disciplined, goal-oriented children with high self-esteem. These techniques have resolved the issues that were chronic sources of anger, anxiety, frustration, and tension in my life, and have made me much happier and healthier than before. I believe they can do the same for you.

In Appendix B you will read letters I have received from those who have recovered rapidly following the recovery plan. I recommend you read Appendix B first, so that you have a better understanding of what the recovery plan can do for you. Appendix C is a guide to all the medical research mentioned in this book. You can use this to discuss with your doctor or health care provider possible changes in your treatment.

Throughout this book I mention other books that I have read about back pain, medicine, health, fitness, communication, stress reduction, and related topics, which will serve as valuable references for you. You will find these books and others in the bibliography.

ADDITIONAL BENEFITS

I should mention here that my increased awareness of the mind/body connection and how tension may manifest itself in a variety of physical symptoms has made a tremendous difference in my health and my life. In addition to the benefits mentioned earlier, you may also benefit in any of the following ways:

1. Require fewer doctor visits
2. Undergo fewer tests and procedures
3. Face less of a chance of improper diagnoses and treatments
4. Endure fewer frustrations and anxieties from dealing with a medical system that ignores your mind and feelings and their effect on your health
5. Reduce or eliminate your need for analgesics, antihistamines, and other medications
6. Save precious time and a great deal of expense
7. Harness your mind's power and abilities to combat pain
8. Aid and utilize your body's own healing system
9. Feel a greater sense of confidence in dealing with your health problems
10. Enjoy better health, and a more enjoyable life because of it

These are some of the many benefits I have experienced since learning more about the mind/body connection—benefits that I will appreciate for the rest of my life. You see, stress and tension are integral parts of our daily lives, and at any age we may face stressful situations that can affect our health; but knowledge of the mind/body connection can help us overcome the physical symptoms more quickly and easily. This awareness also helps us realize how important it is to improve the way we handle stressful situations and relationships. These improvements in turn may help us prevent the more serious health problems associated with tension and stress, such as heart attacks.[16]

So that you get the most out of this book, I want you to set it in your mind right now that you will be among those who recover rapidly and that every step you take from now on will help you achieve this recovery. The more clear you are about what you want to see happen, the more likely you are to achieve it. So take a moment now and set a clear intention in your heart and your mind that every page you read and every step you take will lead you to become pain-free and healthy very soon.

The main purpose and the greatest reward for me in writing this book is to know that you were able to recover from the pain and limitation of disability to live a healthy active life, as a parent, a spouse, a friend, a co-worker, an employer.

I look forward to hearing from those of you who would like to share your experiences and comments. You may write to me care of the publisher:

Health Advisory Group, LLC
2464 El Camino Real, PMB 157
Santa Clara, CA 95051
info@rapidrecovery.net

or e-mail me directly at: fredamir@consultant.com

---

[16] A study published in the *Journal of the American Medical Association,* titled "Effects of Mental Stress on Myocardial Ischemia [chest pain] During Daily Life," concluded: "Mental stress during daily life, including reported feelings of tension, frustration, and sadness, can more than double the risk of myocardial ischemia in the subsequent hour ... and is a significant predictor of future cardiac events" (*JAMA* 277 [May 21, 1997]: 1521–1526).

1

AND THE PAIN BEGAN

STOP *If you skipped the introduction, please stop! The introduction contains some very important information about how this book can help you recover rapidly. Please take a few minutes to read it before going on. Thank you!*

It all began one January morning. At the time I was twenty-nine years old, married, and had two small children. I worked as a registered environmental health specialist for a local health agency in the San Francisco Bay Area.[1] The California Depart-

---

[1] An environmental health specialist is responsible for enforcing state and federal health and safety codes that protect the public health from illnesses caused through improper storage and handling of food, water, sewage, hazardous materials, solid waste, and other environmental factors.

ment of Health Services had just issued emergency regulations regarding hazards associated with the consumption of raw oysters. The oysters harvested from the Gulf of Mexico had been found to contain a salt water bacteria called vibrio vulnificus which, when consumed raw, had caused infections and deaths in susceptible individuals. Those with liver disease, cancer, and other chronic diseases such as diabetes, or conditions that weakened or compromised the immune system, were in danger.

I had been working as an environmental health specialist for more than three years, and I loved my job. Most of my work involved inspecting restaurants, supermarkets, schools, and hospitals to ensure safe and proper storage and handling of food sold and served to the public. I had always believed in the axiom that an ounce of prevention is better than a pound of cure; I did my best to prevent contamination, adulteration, and spoilage of food and food products through educating the owners, managers, and employees of food facilities about the health and safety laws meant to protect the public from food poisoning. Of course, knowledge of safe and proper methods of food handling and good sanitation was not always enough to motivate some operators to observe the law, and sometimes I had to take necessary enforcement actions to obtain compliance. I took pride in my work and felt that each day I was helping to make the world a little safer, even be it in a small way.

When we received the emergency regulations, I quickly determined that about sixty different restaurants, supermarkets, and other retail food facilities in my district were potential sites for selling or serving oysters to their customers. Each of these facilities had to be inspected soon to determine which ones served raw oysters and whether these oysters had been harvested from the Gulf of Mexico.

THE SNAP

I began my investigation by inspecting one facility after another, making frequent stops, getting in and out of the car over and over again. At one of these stops I felt something in my lower back snap as I got out of the car. I ignored it and continued with my investigation. Two weeks later, I woke up to severe pain in my lower back. I had heard of many cases in which back pain was caused by an incident that occurred weeks earlier, so I thought perhaps something in my back had been hurt when I felt the snap. I rested and tried to avoid heavy lifting or any activity that would cause pain, such as carrying my children.

At the time, my daughter was four years old, and my son was two. It was a wonderful time since my son was no longer an infant and had developed the motor skills necessary to allow us to enjoy many more activities together. Our daily routine when I got home from work was to play ring-around-the-rosy or horsey, or to go to the park. I used to combine the fun and games with a few lessons in the alphabet and math to prepare them for their future. But now I was afraid that playing those games could bring on a back-pain attack, and I had to refuse my children's requests to play.

My wife was worried and wanted me to see a doctor. Two years earlier I had had an episode of upper back pain, and my experience with the doctor and physical therapists had not been pleasant. After three months of therapy with no significant improvement, playing soccer twice a week had finally relieved the pain. So I felt now that the best approach to relieve my lower back pain would be to strengthen those muscles on my own, through regular exercise. However, besides a great deal of driving required by my job, I also commuted one hundred miles daily from Concord to San Jose. After putting in twelve to thirteen hours a day commuting and working, I was too tired to exercise regularly; I hoped that when I found us a home near my work, I could begin a daily exercise program.

For nine months I continued to commute, and the pain in my back was tolerable. From time to time it acted up, but for the most part I could ignore it and live a fairly normal life. However, as we prepared to look for a residence close to my work, my wife insisted that I see a doctor so that I would be pain-free by the date we planned to move.

THE GENERAL PRACTITIONER

I went to a general practitioner who had more than twenty-five years of experience. After a brief examination he said there was some muscle strain in my lower back. He prescribed an anti-inflammatory medication, gave me a pamphlet containing a set of back exercises, and said that if I did not improve after a month, he would prescribe physical therapy.

I went home and told my wife that there was nothing to worry about. Later, I tried the exercises in the brochure. For one exercise, known as press-ups, I had to lie on my stomach, keep it on the floor, and press up with my arms as far as I could, bending backwards. According to the instructions, I was supposed to remain in that position for thirty seconds, and gradually build up to five minutes. I did my first press-up and felt pain in my lower back. The pain kept bothering me until I had to lie down and restrict my activities for the rest of the day. I realized that press-ups might not have been the right exercise for my condition.

The next morning I started the commute again. That week I had to work in the hillsides and do a lot of climbing while inspecting construction of a sewage disposal system for a new home. I had to jump over several trenches and felt more pain in my back. By Thursday night it was intolerable. Since I was off on Fridays, I planned to rest and get over this episode of back pain, which I felt was caused by the doctor prescribing the wrong back exercise.

RIGHT-LEG PAIN

When I woke up on Friday morning my right leg was numb, with a great deal of tingling in my right foot. I was in a state of disbelief. I could not understand how this numbness could have come about. I called a friend of mine who had suffered from back and leg pain, and had recently had an operation for a herniated disc. He said that from the description of my symptoms he believed a herniated disc could be a possibility, and he advised me to see a neurosurgeon. I could not understand how I could have developed a herniated disc overnight. And if the press-ups I did were the cause, why it would take four days for the condition to develop? Could the press-ups in combination with climbing hills, jumping over the trenches, and commuting have damaged my spine? I consulted our family encyclopedia on health. It mentioned slipped disc as a cause of leg pain, and bed rest as one of the treatments for it. So, to be on the safe side, I decided to just rest and see whether the pain would improve.

After about three days of rest, my right leg improved, and I was able to walk with much less pain. I did try to see a specialist, but my health plan would not allow me to do so without first being seen by my primary care physician—the same doctor who had given me the exercises that I believed caused the leg pain. I hesitantly made an appointment with my doctor. The doctor did not think that I had a herniated disc, said a pinched nerve was probably causing the leg pain, and did not feel a need for me to see a specialist. When I asked the doctor about the press-ups, he said that I should not have done them. I wondered why he did not tell me that during my first visit.

The doctor ordered an X-ray of my lower back. Later I received a call from his office and was told that the X-ray showed disc degeneration at the L-5 and S-1 vertebrae, and that I had signs of osteoarthritis in my lower back. I had just turned thirty, and the idea that I had developed arthritis in my lower back made me uncomfortable. The word arthritis brought images of old age and disability to my mind. Could it be that all the driving had caused rapid aging in my back?

I took an extra day off and arranged to stay during the week with a friend who lived near my work, so I would not have to commute. The pain in my right leg made it very difficult to climb stairs or walk uphill. After climbing four or five steps, I had to rest a few minutes while the pain subsided, and then climb a few more steps. Also, depending on how severe the stress on my back and legs was, from time to time my left leg also experienced symptoms of pain and tingling. But usually my right leg had the severest symptoms. The leg pain was not only more limiting than an episode of back pain, but also took much longer to improve.

One month later, with the help of friends and relatives, we moved. Shortly afterward, I tried to begin a regular swimming program. Strangely enough, I felt no pain while I swam, but I experienced a lot of pain afterward. Meanwhile, I looked through some books on back pain at the local library. In one, a Harvard University doctor described any back pain older than four weeks as chronic and hard to treat. He also mentioned that freeway driving causes disc degeneration.

I became worried. All the freeway driving I had done must have damaged my back, and now that my injury was chronic, I thought, it would be hard to treat. However, I was not commuting anymore and was pain-free most of the time; I hoped the damage was not that great and that strengthening my back muscles would prevent further damage.

WORKERS' COMPENSATION

After about two months I had another attack of low back pain and right leg pain. I decided I needed professional help and went to see a family doctor in a well-respected medical group. His examination revealed lower back muscle strain and possibly a pinched nerve causing my leg pain, for which he prescribed anti-inflammatory medication, a muscle relaxant, and physical therapy. For a number of reasons—one of them being the impact on my career—I had made no mention of my back pain at work so far. However, it was becoming increasingly difficult for me to work in hilly areas, so I decided to file for workers' compensation and have my job responsibilities modified to accommodate my condition. Another reason I filed a claim was that I thought my employer, like many others, would refer me to doctors and therapists who usually take care of employees with back problems, and that I would thereby avoid improper medical treatment. Unfortunately, my employer's program left the choice of doctors and therapists to me. Since mine was a case of muscle strain and the pain usually improved with rest, I thought all that I needed was a few sessions of physical therapy.

PHYSICAL THERAPY

The therapist treated me with heat, ultrasound, massage, stretching, and interferential (electrical) stimulation. I was told that heat and ultrasound help increase blood flow to the area and speed healing, and the interferential stimulation somehow confuses the mind and reduces its perception of pain. I was also given a set of stretches to do at home. These were very effective; as soon as I felt some pain, I performed the stretches and the pain went away. In fact, after one week of physical therapy I became almost pain-free.

However, as my episodes of back pain became less frequent, I noticed a very painful swelling in my gum, but could not figure out how I got it. Instead of ignoring it the way I did my back pain, I decided to be on the safe side and have it checked. I went to see my dentist and got caught in the Friday afternoon traffic jam, turning a twenty-minute drive into a very frustrating fifty-minute one. The dentist checked my gum and said that I might have hit something on it to cause the swelling, but that it didn't appear serious. The next morning, however, I woke up with severe pain in my lower back. I was really surprised, because my back had been doing much better. The previous day's drive had been frustrating, but it wasn't any worse than driving one hundred miles daily, which I had done before for so many months without experiencing so much pain. I did the stretches, but this time they did not help. Fortunately this episode happened on a weekend, and after two days of rest I was well enough to return to work on Monday.

I went to therapy for another three weeks, but the same pattern continued. Something would happen on Friday or Saturday to cause me back and leg pain, and by Monday I would be well enough to go to work. Unfortunately, the therapy group I went to was very busy, and different therapists took care of me on almost every visit, which made for an inconsistent treatment program. The one who spent the most time on my case told me that I should feel some pain when I stretched. So I stretched to the point of feeling pain, and as a result strained my muscles. When I began the more advanced therapy program, I ended up with more pain, especially more leg pain, or sciatica. (The sciatic nerve goes down the legs from the back; pain or any discomfort associated with that nerve is called sciatica.)

POOL THERAPY

After more than a month of physical therapy, I had to take two weeks off to recover from it! My back and leg pain improved during those two weeks, after which I began a pool therapy program to strengthen my back muscles. There I met patients who had been diagnosed with herniated discs but were told by their doctors to try pool therapy first. If the pool therapy did not eliminate the pain, they were to have surgery. Apparently surgery is no longer the first option when it comes to back pain; more conservative approaches are tried first. I wondered why walking in water and strengthening back muscles would eliminate pain caused by a herniated disc pressing on the nerve. Some who had had surgery despite the pool therapy were now back for more therapy, since the surgery had not eliminated their pain. The experiences of these people made me more puzzled about the diagnosis and treatment of back pain. I also discovered that the patients I met had disc abnormalities at the lower, L4-L5 and L5-S1 vertebrae, and I wondered what makes the lower part of the spine so vulnerable.

Some of the other patients I met had tried chiropractic manipulations, acupuncture, massage therapy, ice or heat packs, ointments, and oriental herbal teas to relieve their pain. These treatments had temporarily alleviated pain. I had found the cooling pain-relief ointments and ice massage worked well for me. But, like all other such treatments, the relief was only temporary.

The pool therapy worked for a while. I was able to stop taking the anti-inflammatory medication and felt some improvement. But when I had to stay in the office one day and sit for an extended period of time, I experienced severe pain in my leg that night. I had been free of sciatic pain for about three weeks at that time. This recurrence surprised me because I had done office duty before without experiencing any problem. I realized that certain things I used to do before were going to cause me a lot of pain if I did them now. But it was difficult to know in advance what these things were, so I had to become more and more careful and avoid positions or activities that might cause pain later.[2]

My social life became very limited because sitting more than fifteen or twenty minutes caused sciatica that took several days to improve. It was difficult to invite friends to our home because I was uncomfortable unless I could lie down, something I was embarrassed about doing in front of visitors. I was in no condition to visit friends, either; I certainly didn't want to go to their homes and lie down. I also discovered how difficult it is for most people to deal with someone in chronic pain. Many of my friends had expected me to recover in a couple of weeks. When this expectation was not fulfilled, many of them reduced and eventually discontinued their contact with me. I was quite surprised to see how quickly they gave up on me. Of course, I was not too eager to call anyone, because the first thing my friends asked about was my back, and I did not care to make my condition the main topic of conversation. I came to the painful realization that the limits on my abilities meant the loss of many friends.[3] This lack of social life was very difficult, especially for my wife and children.

My physical limitations had also increased. Now carrying anything heavier than five pounds would cause sciatica. My right leg and buttock were so sensitive that I had to wear shoes whenever I walked and sit on a foam cushion. I felt guilty because I was unable to play with my children as I used to. They wanted me to hold them, carry them, and play ring-around-the-rosy, horsey, and all the other games I used to play with them. Sometimes they came to me crying, asking whether I would ever get well. My

---

[2] In the next few months, as the list of positions and movements that might cause pain grew, I became more and more limited in my abilities and mobility.

[3] Julie Zimmerman, a physical therapist, in her book *Chronic Back Pain: Moving On*, provides an excellent account of how chronic back pain affects the person's social life. (Brunswick, Maine: Biddle Publishing, 1991, pp. 47–50).

limited ability to help with the children and other obligations at home placed added stress on my wife, who was already quite worried about me.

I felt guilty that I had not taken this problem seriously from the start; I should not have ignored the pain for so long and commuted so much. If I had sought treatment right away, perhaps my disc would not have degenerated so much and this wouldn't have become such a frustrating problem. I lived in constant fear of damaging my spine further.

THE SEARCH

About this time, a friend gave me a book on proper back care and good body mechanics, written by the director of a back institute. The author conducts training seminars for various companies. This book explained that proper stretching should not involve pain, which made me wonder how a registered physical therapist could have misled me on such a simple yet crucial point. Reading the book made me realize that I had to take an active role in my treatment; otherwise I could be seriously hurt by the people who were supposed to help me. The book also discussed how various positions and movements put pressure on the spine and how using proper body mechanics in daily activities can reduce that pressure to a minimum. Putting these techniques into practice really helped take pressure off my back, and consequently I experienced very little back pain.[4]

NECK PAIN

Now, however, I began to have pain in the right side of my neck. It started suddenly: one morning, it was very difficult and painful to turn my neck. I applied ice and began to do some of the stretches mentioned in the book on body mechanics, and I talked

---

[4] The author did, however, point out that even if one becomes an expert in good body mechanics, there are times when one can still suffer from back pain for no apparent reason!

to my physical therapist. She told me that it is very common for people with back problems to also develop neck pain. After a few days of doing the stretches the pain subsided, but my neck remained very sensitive—so sensitive that I could no longer wear a tie. As a government official, I had always tried my best to be presentable and wear formal clothing. Now, even my choice of clothing had become limited.

THE ORTHOPEDIC SURGEON

The really frustrating thing, however, was the sciatica, which would by no means go away. At times my right leg became so stiff that I could barely bend it and had to limp most of the time; my right foot felt as heavy as a cement block and sometimes very cold. After a few days, when the sciatica improved, the pain concentrated in my upper buttock area. The book on back pain had been very helpful, so I decided to contact the author at her institute and see what solution she might have for sciatica. She recommended that I see a highly respected, nationally known orthopedic surgeon who was her close family friend and practiced in the Bay Area. She was so nice as to offer to call the doctor's office personally if I could not get an appointment sometime soon.

I was able to get an appointment for two weeks later, but continued my search. I came across a book called *The Diagnosis and Misdiagnosis of Back Pain* by Julie Zimmerman, herself a physical therapist who had suffered for years from chronic back pain.[5] In her book she explained that the piriformis syndrome can

---

[5] In the preface to her book, Ms. Zimmerman writes about her search for a cure and the many doctors and treatments she tried. She was seen by her family doctor, an orthopedic surgeon, a neurologist, a neurosurgeon, a rheumatologist, two osteopaths, an acupuncturist, and two physical therapists. She tried a number of physical treatments as well as positive thinking. She was given a number of different diagnoses for her condition but was left with "low back pain" as her official diagnosis. She was eventually told by her doctor that her disability was probably permanent and that she would have to learn to live with it.

be one cause of sciatica. The piriformis is a muscle located in the upper buttock area whose job is to help rotate the hip, and in some people the sciatic nerve apparently passes near or right through this muscle. That was exactly where my pain concentrated, in the upper part of my buttock. Sciatica is caused by the sciatic nerve becoming compressed due to a spasm of the piriformis muscle. The piriformis goes into spasm in an attempt to stabilize the area due to stress on the lumbar region of the spine. Ms. Zimmerman listed a number of usual treatments: electrical stimulation, massage, stretching the muscle, steroid injection, and surgically cutting the muscle.[6] I also found the same syndrome mentioned in Dr. Rene Calliet's book *Low Back Pain Syndrome*.[7] However, the only treatment he suggested was a steroid (cortisone) injection into the muscle, without mentioning other, noninvasive treatments.

I was very happy to finally find a plausible explanation for the source of sciatica and pain in my upper buttock: stress placed on the piriformis muscle caused it to go into spasm and pinch the nerve every time I sat too long or carried objects weighing more than five pounds. So I began to stretch the piriformis, and gradually it began to put less and less stress on my sciatic nerve. After a few days the sciatica was gone. I was able to walk without a limp and was beginning to feel that after so many weeks I was actually on my way to full recovery. I postponed my appointment with the orthopedic surgeon for two weeks.

About this time, my parents came for a surprise visit. They were happy about my improvement. We had a barbecue and went out for a short drive. When we came home, all of a sudden both my legs went into severe spasm. *What is it this time?* I wondered.

---

[6] Zimmerman, Julie, *The Diagnosis and Misdiagnosis of Back Pain*, pp.111–114. According to Dr. Loren Fishman, in some cases even surgery does not relieve the symptoms (Brody, Jane E., "The Roots of Sciatica Aren't Always Linked to Back Problems," *New York Times*, April 15, 1992).

[7] Calliet, Rene, M.D., *Low Back Pain Syndrome* (4th ed.) (Philadelphia: F. A. Davis, 1988), pp. 280–282.

Why both legs? I put ice on them and did some stretching. I kept thinking, *What could have happened now?*

By the next day the spasms started to get better. There was no sciatica, but now both piriformis muscles were in severe pain. After some thinking, I realized that the three leg raises I had done the night before had been a little difficult. Probably that, in combination with helping out with the barbecue and taking my parents out, was too much for my muscles.

After a few days of increased mobility, I had to spend another frustrating weekend in bed. This time my daughter, who was five at the time, came to me crying, "Daddy, are you ever going to get well?" I really did not know what to tell her. Before this latest setback, I had planned to cancel my appointment with the orthopedic surgeon, to try a much more conservative exercise program, and to hope that my condition would, as it had done earlier, begin to improve. But when my little girl came to me with her beautiful eyes filled with tears, I felt that maybe going to this doctor, a nationally known orthopedic surgeon, would help. After all, it was now fourteen months since my back pain had begun.

THE MRI

Eventually, I was seen by the orthopedic surgeon and his associate. He listened to a brief history of my case, and without even doing an examination insisted that I must have an MRI. MRI stands for magnetic resonance imaging, which unlike the X-ray produces images of soft tissues, such as a disc, allowing the detection of a herniated disc. I explained to the surgeon that I had been able to eliminate the pain in my right leg by stretching the piriformis muscle and did not believe that the pain was disc-related. His response was that my right sciatic nerve was probably pinched in two locations, at the piriformis muscle and somewhere else that could involve a herniated disc. He told me that the only way to find out for sure would be through an MRI. I was hesitant, and asked for an explanation. "If the disc is herniated, why isn't the sciatic pain constant, and how come I'd been able to eliminate it by stretching the piriformis?" I wondered aloud.

At that point, seeing that he had not yet convinced me, this gray-haired gentleman put his hand on my shoulder and in a very fatherly manner said that this recommendation was based on his years of experience dealing with thousands of back patients. He added that just as it would be foolish for him to claim expertise in environmental health, it would be foolish for me to act as my own doctor.

Now I had to make a decision between trusting my own diagnosis, based on the few books I had read on back pain, or relying on the judgment of a nationally known and highly respected orthopedic surgeon with years of experience. Naturally, I opted for the latter, and I decided to have the MRI done. The doctor left my examination to his associate, who diagnosed me as having herniated nucleus pulposus of the lumbar spine (herniated disc), clinical facet syndrome, and possible piriformis syndrome.[8] The MRI was scheduled for the following week.

By now my piriformis muscles had become less painful and I had no sciatica. I thought perhaps if I felt better by next week I might postpone the MRI. But unfortunately, about this time I came down with a rash. I thought it might have been due to a change in our detergent. I checked out two books from the library on skin care, and both mentioned allergic reaction as one cause of a rash. However, the cause of most rashes is still a mystery.[9] The rash was so severe that I had to take a whole week off from work. It was very uncomfortable. I could not wear any tight clothing. I was prescribed a cortisone lotion and recovered after about a week, just in time for the MRI. This chain of events, of course, matched the usual pattern. As soon as one problem began to improve, something else happened to hinder my recovery.

---

[8] Despite the fact that he did not conduct an examination, the orthopedic surgeon wrote down in my chart that it sounded to him that I had a disc problem and might need surgery. Regarding our discussion he wrote, "The patient has clearly studied considerable information about his symptoms and feels he has piriformis syndrome."

[9] Walzer, Richard, M.D., *Healthy Skin: A Guide for Life Long Skin Care* (Mt. Vernon, N.Y.: Consumer Union, 1989).

THE SHOT

I had the MRI done. The scan showed a marked degeneration at the L5-S1 vertebrae, and desiccation and annular deformity at L4-5 with bulging; the diagnosis was protrusion degeneration at L4-5 and L5-S1 and piriformis syndrome. But there was no evidence of disc herniation.

I was seen by the internist, who explained that there was no need for surgery. I asked him what the best treatment would be. He said that a piriformis block, a steroid (cortisone) shot into the muscle, would definitely help me.

"Are you sure, Doctor, since I have not had sciatica for a month now, that this would really help?" I asked.

He said, "Oh, yes." I asked him again whether the shot would be the best treatment and explained to him that I was scheduled to start a more advanced physical therapy program on Monday. He assured me there should be no problem with the physical therapy program, and that the shot would take care of all the recurring problems I had had. In fact, he was so positive about the shot that I joked with him about playing soccer the next day. He joked back, saying, "Well, maybe not soccer, but you might want to go skydiving."

As I left to go to the section where I would receive the shot under X- ray, I thought it might be a good idea to delay it a week so I could read more about it. However, I decided that at some point I needed to trust a doctor with my treatment. After all, this was a well-known clinic dedicated to back problems.

I was given the shot along with a pain-killing agent, so I didn't feel any pain when the 3½-inch needle was stuck into my piriformis muscle, but as soon as the effects of the painkiller wore off, my sciatica started. I began to feel severe pain in the piriformis and was really surprised. I asked the nurse, "Am I supposed to feel so much pain?" The nurse said, "Oh, yes. You mean your doctor hasn't prescribed any pain medication?" I thought to myself, *Pain medication!* She added that it would take three to four days minimum for the pain caused by the steroid shot to go away. I could not believe that the doctor had made it sound so painless and joked to me about going skydiving the next day. The only good thing was that I received the shot on a Friday afternoon. I hoped that by Monday I would be well enough to go back to work.

That night I was unable to fall asleep because of the pain. I had to take some Tylenol PM, which helped relieve the pain a little so I could get some sleep. I was really upset about what had happened, and all the undue pain that I was caused by this so-called back specialist. How could he mislead me in such a way? I felt betrayed.[10]

The next day when I woke up I had severe hiccups, upset stomach, and severe pain in the piriformis muscle and in my lower back. I was just getting over a whole week of restricted activity due to the rash, and now this! I called the surgeon's office; the doctor on call said: "There's nothing to worry about. As the pain gets better, you can begin physical therapy."

By Sunday my stomach was less irritated, and my hiccups were gone, but I was still in pain and frustrated. I was not sure about beginning advanced physical therapy while I was in pain. On Monday I tried to contact the orthopedic surgeon for advice, but I was told that his policy was not to speak to any patients on the phone, which made me more frustrated.

After about three days I was in less pain and decided doing some minor stretches might help. But the little stretching that I did, as carefully as I could, brought back the sciatica later that night. Now I was very upset. I had no appetite. I had trouble breathing and could take only shallow breaths. I went back to my family doctor the next day. He was not a back specialist, but I

---

[10] Usually I would forgive and forget such incidents, but no more. I have learned the hard way to stand up for my medical rights. I filed complaints with every medical association I could think of and the California State Medical Board. The county medical association investigated the case and condemned the internist's conduct. Unfortunately, such condemnations amount to no more than a slap on the wrist, and such cases are not considered serious enough for a malpractice suit.

knew he would not hurt me. He listened to me carefully and checked me for other symptoms. "You know, I think you have been under a lot of stress. Just take things easy and you'll be fine," he told me at the end of a forty-five minute visit.

I will never forget this visit and the time he spent carefully listening to me and evaluating my condition, for which I will be always grateful to him. Indeed, a caring doctor can make a world of difference in patients' lives; I felt a lot better after our conversation. My appetite improved, and my breathing returned to normal.

After a few days I began the pool therapy. Walking in the water seemed to be the only thing that helped. I had to stop all stretching, because every time I stretched the sciatic nerve acted up. One of the therapists had told me that if I used the muscle and tired it by walking in water, it would help the muscle to relax and not press on the nerve. After doing that for about two weeks, I noticed some improvement. I could sit and walk longer without much discomfort. I felt that this time I was really improving. However, this much improvement was too good to be true. After those two weeks of improvement, I woke up one morning with a hoarse voice and coughing. That night after the pool therapy, I got home and came down with a fever of 104°F. It was bronchitis. Later the bronchitis developed into pneumonia, and I ended up being off work for two weeks.

Finally, after two weeks of rest, on Saturday I was going to go back to walking in the pool. But I woke up with severe pain in the right side of my abdomen. I thought it must be my appendix. I could barely breathe or walk from the pain. My wife rushed me to the doctor. He could not find any physical indication for the pain and thought it might be muscle strain. I attributed it to putting my son on my lap the night before, although I had done so many times before while sitting down without causing myself any pain. Why would doing the same thing cause pain this time? And why would the pain begin the next day? I did not know. The only explanation seemed to be that my muscles were weakened due to my long period of restricted activity, so that the slightest exertion led to strain. The doctor prescribed some painkillers, and after a week I was able to return to work.

These were trying times. I seemed to be trapped in a vicious cycle of pain and illness with no end in sight. As soon as one thing improved, something else happened to me. However, I saw it as a test and believed all this was happening due to a purpose. I thanked God for all the blessings I had been given, especially for my two beautiful, healthy children, and focused on the positive aspects of my life. After all, many people were in worse condition and much more pain than I. I reminded myself how difficult it must be for people who have a recurrence of cancer and have to go through chemotherapy again.

THE SEARCH CONTINUES

As I continued my search for an answer, I came across a book entitled *Backache Relief,* a survey of nearly five hundred back patients done by two *New York Times* writers.[11] According to the survey, anyone, at any time, could suffer from back pain. One survey participant was a forty-five-year-old man who ran ten miles daily, did fifty sit-ups, practiced yoga, and was quite limber. Yet even he suffered from back pain for more than four years.

The book pointed out the difficulties back patients face in finding proper care. It included an amazing list of more than twenty back specialists, ranging from orthopedists to shiatsu therapists,[12] from whom the patients surveyed in the book had sought help. Each practitioner had his or her own particular bias and terminology in diagnosing the source of the pain and recommending treatment. Needless to say, for the same back pain, patients were given a different diagnosis by each "specialist." Seeking treatment for my back pain increasingly seemed like

---

[11] Klien, Arthur, and Sobel, Dava, *Backache Relief* (New York: Penguin Books, 1985).

[12] Shiatsu therapy is a form of massage therapy that uses acupressure to relieve pain (Klien and Sobel, p. 68).

wandering through a great big maze with no apparent way out.

The survey also included interviews with patients who had suffered from sciatica, some for more than twenty years. Reading these interviews made me realize that I might be in this condition for many years to come. The book recommended avoiding orthopedists, general practitioners, and neurosurgeons for sciatica, as these practitioners had apparently made the patients who were surveyed feel worse. The book also advised that if you have the slightest doubt about your doctor, even if he or she is the most respected doctor in the world, make sure that you get out of that office and never go back, because wrong treatment could make you worse. In fact, many of the back patients were given the wrong set of back exercises by one doctor or another and as a result had become worse. I felt relieved to know that I was not the only one having difficulty finding proper medical care. After the experiences I had had with some of my doctors, I was beginning to wonder if it was just me.

The book provided suggestions on how to deal with sciatica and which medical practitioners would be helpful.[13] Apparently a good physical therapist and a doctor of physical medicine (physiatrist) had been of great help to many patients suffering from sciatica. So I decided to see a physiatrist. To find the best ones in my area I surveyed fifteen different physical therapy groups by phone; two physiatrists were highly recommended by most of them. They both worked in the same industrial medicine clinic.

THE PHYSIATRIST

This time, after I made an appointment, I prepared a set of questions to ask the doctor in order to evaluate his knowledge and responsiveness to my concerns. After reading *Backache Relief,* I had learned much more about back specialists and what to expect.

Eventually I was seen by one of the two physiatrists. He was very responsive to my questions, very courteous, and appeared

---

[13] Klien and Sobel, pp. 310-319.

disturbed about the cortisone shot that I had received. He attributed the sciatica to fluid inside the disc leaking out and irritating the nerve. This he felt was also the reason that I experienced a delayed worsening of the pain and sciatica due to activities such as standing or sitting longer than usual. Then he referred me to a very competent and experienced physical therapist. The therapist spent more than an hour asking me questions and trying to see how well I used body mechanics. He was very thorough and appeared quite concerned. I felt good about both of these visits.

By now it was July and I had made arrangements for a two-day family vacation in Monterey. My son, who was three at the time, had come up to me a few weeks earlier and asked, "Daddy, are we going on vacation this year?" And then he had immediately said, "Oh, we can't, because your back hurts so much." I felt so bad. My pain and disability had been very hard on him. So hard that, during a visit to his aunt's house in Concord, he had asked her and her husband whether he could live with them as their second son. I already felt quite inadequate as it was, and hearing him ask this question certainly made me feel even worse, as my wish to be a good husband and father seemed harder and harder to realize.

So when my son mentioned the vacation, I decided that no matter how much pain it was going to cause me, we had to go on this vacation. And so we did. The drive to Monterey was an hour and a half long. I lay down in the back seat of our van; we stopped after forty-five minutes so I could get out of the van and walk around a little in order to relieve the pain. During our stay in Monterey, I would lie in the van and my wife would take the kids on the carousel, or to the parks, or for a boat ride. I could not join them, but just the knowledge that they were enjoying themselves was very satisfying to me. To my great surprise, when we came back, my right leg was much better. I thought that possibly this improvement was due to the way I had positioned my leg in the van; the muscle was under much less stress, and that had probably helped.

I began therapy with the new physical therapist, and we tried a number of different stretches. However, the sciatica became severe again, and my right leg would become so stiff that I could not bend it. I was quite worried about permanent nerve damage and loss of sensation and strength in my right leg. Some of the readings I had done had mentioned this outcome as a possibility. So I decided to stop all physical therapy for a while and do the only thing that seemed to work: walking in the pool. Besides its physical benefits, this activity also seemed very comforting and invigorating to me.

LEFT-LEG PAIN

It was clear from the pattern of the past few months that if I didn't develop more pain in my back or leg, I would come down with neck pain, rash, or some other ailment. It was clear to me and my wife that it was only a matter of time before I would be unable to work. So we decided to move to a more affordable residence, as we were renting a house at the time. In the course of looking for an apartment, I walked up a stairway faster than usual, relying mainly on my left leg; I didn't want the apartment manager to know I had a physical problem. Shortly after, I felt pain in the left groin area. To be on the safe side, I rested that Saturday and put ice on the affected area.

Sunday I felt well. There was no pain. So I went back to the pool. The next day, at four in the morning, my son woke up coughing. I gave him some cough medication and went back to sleep. When I got up at 5:30 a.m. to go to work, I realized that my left leg was irritated. It seemed very strange, because this time it wasn't the sciatic nerve that goes down the back of the buttock and leg that hurt, it was on the inside of my left leg. It also seemed strange that I was fine at 4:00 a.m. but only an hour and a half later woke up with an irritated nerve in my left leg.

What could have happened? I thought that perhaps I had injured myself on Saturday by going up the stairs, and probably walking in the pool had contributed to worsening the inflammation. I decided to take that day off from work and rest. From past experience, I had learned that there were times when electrical stimulation had helped to quiet down the nerve, so I thought that it would be a good idea to go to physical therapy and have that done.

I called my therapist, and he fit me in at about 5:30 that afternoon. By then my left leg was better. I went in hoping that the electrical stimulation would help relieve the symptoms faster and I would be able to go back to work the next day. He explained to me that the sciatic nerve also runs on the inside of the leg. So now I had sciatica in my left leg as well. The therapist's staff used heat, some massage, and the electrical stimulant on my leg. But about half an hour later I experienced the most severe sciatic pain ever. It was intolerable. I began taking anti-inflammatory medication, but it did not help. So I took a painkiller. The combination of the anti-inflammatory medication and the painkiller caused dizziness and disorientation. I called the physiatrist; he prescribed a steroid medication that did not help much either. I could not sleep at night because of the pain.

I was very angry at myself, first for going up the stairs, which I felt I should not have done in the first place; and because I did my pool exercise the next day, instead of waiting three or four days, and thereby possibly worsened the inflammation. And then, again, I made the mistake of going back to the therapist thinking that therapy would help. In my case, it seemed every time I went to the therapist, I got worse. I tried to comfort myself by reminding myself that when one is in pain and frustrated, looking for a quick solution is natural, and it is easy to make such mistakes. And it seemed to me that I would have gotten worse anyway, even if I hadn't done anything! I stayed off work three days, until I could tolerate standing and sitting in one position long enough to carry out my duties. My left leg was so sensitive that even my pants rubbing on my skin bothered me.

With sciatica in both legs my life had now become more and more restricted. I needed to rest more often. I had a very difficult time standing in one position for more than ten minutes. I had to shift around more often. It was becoming increasingly difficult to carry out my duties at work. I had already had difficulty attending staff meetings, training seminars, and other events and situations that required sitting or standing longer than twenty minutes, but now taking part in such activities became impossible. I had to delay inspection of sites that were too hard for me to visit due to the presence of a stairway or conditions that involved walking over 100 feet continuously. When necessary I would ask one of my colleagues to do such an inspection for me. I often had to take part of a day off due to pain, so that I gradually lost the little vacation time I had accrued (fortunately, I had a caring supervisor who tried to accommodate my condition). At home, I could no longer stand in one position long enough to wash the dishes or be helpful to my wife and children. The little that I could do before was no longer possible.

2

NOT THE KNEES!

*T*hree weeks after the problem with my left leg began, I started to feel pain in my left knee. I attributed the pain to my having put too much pressure on my left leg and knee while climbing the apartment stairs. So now I had to rely more on the right leg. In a way, this change was funny, because the right leg had been the bad leg for a long time, but now, compared to the left leg, it was much better. Gradually, my right knee started to bother me as well. Whenever I stepped up onto a curb, my right knee hurt. It also felt irritated whenever I sat down awhile. So, as usual, I went to the library and checked out a couple of books on knee health. My problem seemed to be a case of chondromalacia patella.[1]

I had never had knee pain before. Because knee problems can involve tendons and ligaments, I became concerned about serious structural damage and went to see my physical therapist for a diagnosis. He said, "It's tendinitis." I had been limping all the time because of sciatica in both legs, which put a lot of pressure on my knees, thus causing the tendinitis. He strongly advised me to stay home from work the rest of the week and take anti-inflammatory medication to speed up my recovery.

---

[1] Chondromalacia patella is a roughening of the underside of the patella (kneecap).

GASTRITIS

That advice would have been fine, except that a week earlier I had developed gastritis. My stomach was feeling very irritated and hurt when I ate. My own doctor was on vacation. The doctor covering for him examined me and said, "Due to all the anti-inflammatory medication you have taken, you might have developed an ulcer." The stool sample he tested was negative, but he said that he wanted an upper GI series done, which involved a series of X-rays of the stomach. It seemed strange that even though there was no blood in the stool, the doctor still seemed to think that I might have an ulcer and wanted to order an upper GI series.

Being on the conservative side when it comes to medications and X-rays, and also not knowing this doctor and how careful he was, I went to the library and checked out a couple of books on gastrointestinal health. One of them, *Gastrointestinal Health* by Dr. Steven Peikin, explained that it is quite common for patients who take anti-inflammatory medications to develop an inflammation of the stomach lining known as gastritis.[2] One symptom of gastritis is that eating aggravates the condition. The same medication given for ulcer is also used to treat gastritis.

When I read this explanation, of course, I realized that probably my problem was gastritis. This conclusion seemed especially likely since eating irritated my stomach, whereas eating relieves ulcer pain by neutralizing stomach acid. I had a prescription from my own doctor for a blood test. I had my blood tested, and all the counts were normal, which meant I was not bleeding internally. In any case, the same treatment is used for both gastritis and ulcer. So I started taking Zantac, which reduces stomach acid, so that my stomach would have a chance to heal. When my doctor came back from vacation, I consulted him by phone. He agreed with my diagnosis, and saw no reason that I should need a series of X-rays.

---

[2] Steven Peikin, M.D., *Gastrointestinal Health* (New York: Harper-Collins, 1991), pp. 41–42.

Here again the first doctor who examined me did not hesitate to order a series of X-rays, paying no attention to my symptoms or to the test that he himself conducted in his office. There was no blood in the stool, and eating increased my pain; so why should the doctor assume that I might have an ulcer? In contrast, my own doctor, a careful, caring man, diagnosed my problem as gastritis. This incident reinforced for me the importance of reading and learning as much as possible about our illnesses and their treatments. That information can save money, time, trouble, and a considerable amount of pain.

An irritated stomach forced new limitations on me. I could not drink orange juice or eat foods with tomato sauce in them. Whenever I got upset, my stomach became irritated. It was so sensitive that it would become irritated when I so much as looked at an orange.

OFF WORK

Nineteen months after my back pain began, on the advice of the physical therapist and my family doctor I decided to take time off from work and rest. I had read enough to know that staying home and bed rest could make matters worse. It is better to keep moving and remain active to prevent other physical problems, such as loss of muscle strength due to inactivity. I had been trying to remain active since my back pain began. However, with knee problems I didn't want to take the chance of causing some serious structural damage. I thought it would be best to be seen by the physiatrist I had dealt with before, but he had moved on to another clinic. I made an appointment with the other highly recommended physiatrist. My physical therapist had also worked with this physiatrist and considered him to be very competent. I managed to make an appointment with him a week later.

THE SECOND PHYSIATRIST

At the clinic the physiatrist conducted a brief examination and was quite surprised and very upset to learn that I had been given a steroid shot in my piriformis muscle. I said to myself, *Well, that's a good sign. At least he is willing to criticize another doctor openly.* But then he discredited the idea that the piriformis muscle could be the source of the sciatic problem. He insisted that I undergo electromyography (EMG), which involves sticking needles in the muscles to measure electrical activity. An abnormal pattern of activity may indicate muscle disease or nerve impairment. I had read in the book *Backache Relief* that most of those who had an EMG had found it not to be helpful in any way, and some of them had found it a very painful test. I tried to have an intelligent discussion with the doctor. "Could you explain to me why I would need this test?" I asked.

He said, "Well, you've had this problem for a long time, and I think this test would really show us what we need to do."

I said, "As far as I understand, the test basically shows the possible location of a pinched nerve. So could you explain to me what kind of treatment I can expect? Let's say you find that a certain muscle in my thigh, for example, is pinching on the nerve. What would the treatment be?"

His arrogant response was, "I do not have the time to explain these things to you right now."[3]

I said, "Well, if you do not have the time to explain the treatment options to me, I don't see any reason why I should have an EMG done."

To this he said, "There are certain medications we can give, certain shots, stretches, and exercises that can be done, but that will be determined after the test."

By now, of course, I had read enough to know there is no

---

[3] In the words of John Steinbeck, "The medical profession is unconsciously irritated by lay knowledge" (quoted in *Medicine on Trial: The Appalling Story of Ineptitude, Malfeasance, Neglect, and Arrogance,* by Charles B. Inlander, president of People's Medical Society [Englewood Cliffs, N.J.: Prentice-Hall, 1988], p.18). Inlander has coauthored a number of valuable books on the medical establishment, among them *Your Medical Rights* and *Take This Book to The Hospital with You.*

magic cure for back pain or sciatica, and I saw no point in having the test. I told the doctor, "I'd like to wait a month and if I'm not better, then maybe at that time I'll have an EMG done."

He stated his displeasure with my decision and added, "I cannot give you a note to stay off work for a month. I hope you understand that."

I said, "Oh, well, that's fine." I had already obtained a note from my family doctor for staying off work, so I didn't have to worry about his threat of making me return to work in pain.

Then he said, "You know, let me check something." And he began to examine me once more. He pressed on my discs, piriformis muscles, and legs so hard that I was in pain for an entire week—as if he wanted to punish me for not accepting his decision.

I was furious at him and at myself. I should have known by that time not to go to another back specialist, no matter how highly recommended. How could such doctors be allowed to practice medicine? I even called the district attorney's office to file a complaint. I was told that it was the doctor's word against mine and that I did not have a winnable case.

ELBOW PAIN

Now I was home resting, occasionally going out to the therapist's or to the pool. I was in pain most of the time and had to change positions constantly from lying down to sitting to walking; otherwise, the pain and irritation would get worse. Meanwhile I mainly relied on my upper body strength any time I had to get up and move about from a sitting or lying position. After about four weeks I began to feel pain in my elbows. The therapist showed me some stretches for the elbows and exercises such as wall push-ups. My elbows improved a little, but now I began to have pain in my wrists!

A few days later, during a follow-up visit, my family doctor examined my elbows and asked, "Do your hands feel numb at night?" I answered, "No, not yet, but the way things have been going, that may be next." And, sure enough, a couple of nights later, I began to have problems with my forearm and hands becoming numb and waking me up in the middle of the night. This experience—waking up unable to feel my hands—was really scary.

SEVERELY DISABLED

Now, with my elbows and wrists in pain, it was becoming more and more difficult to take care of myself. This was the hardest of all the physical limitations I had experienced. Before, in spite of the back and leg pain, I could somehow go where I had to and get things done. Now I had to hold a cup of water with both hands to bring it to my mouth for a drink, and even that effort caused a great deal of pain. I could get a one-quart container of milk out of the refrigerator only with difficulty; a half-gallon container was impossible for me to lift. Pouring juice into a glass took quite a bit of maneuvering. Besides not being able to pick things up off the floor, now I had to ask for help when reaching up for things because of the pain in my elbows.

I could no longer hold a book while lying down. At least before, when I lay down to rest, I could hold a book and read it, but that was no longer possible. I found even writing two lines very painful. The pain in my elbows and hands restricted my activity to a far greater extent than anything I had experienced before. I was beginning to develop some sense of what it meant to be almost totally disabled and dependent on others. My body was becoming a prison for my mind. I thought to myself, *If I ever recover from this, I have indeed experienced a level of disability that very few people do in their entire life.* And what a feeling it would be to live a pain-free, able life again!

I had now become so limited that my wife had to do everything. In addition to her daily eighty-mile commute and work, she also did everything around the house, from taking care of the children and me to doing the laundry and washing the dishes. I felt sorry for her and guilty about my inability to help her. It was a very difficult time for her.

"It's All in Your Head"

One of the funny things about what I was experiencing was all the advice I was given by well-meaning friends and relatives. This advice ranged from the suggestion that eating a lot of shrimp would cure me, to a command to ignore my pain and go for a regular five-mile jog. I also heard every chronic pain sufferer's favorite: "It's all in your head. Just don't think about it and you'll be fine." Actually, I had tried to ignore the pain and sit longer than usual, or walk without a limp, but every time I did so the pain and irritation came back with a vengeance. I had even read a book about relieving back pain using acupressure and meditation. These techniques brought some temporary relief, but I thought these methods simply masked the problem rather than curing it.

It was also suggested to me to see a neurologist, chiropractor, or other "back specialist." My wife thought that I might have developed some kind of joint disease and that I should see a rheumatologist. My response to the idea of seeing another specialist dealing with back pain was that they would probably want to run more tests to make some other diagnosis and make more money, and I would get worse in the process. Most of the so-called experts I had consulted were either unwilling or unable to provide a reasonable explanation for my questions, so how could I expect a cure from them? As far as I was concerned, as chronic and limiting as my condition was, it could not be as serious as it appeared.

To me, this evaluation of my condition was simply common sense. After all, I had not been in a serious car accident or contracted some strange disease. As far as I knew I suffered from a combination of some weak muscles and stressed tendons, and I should eventually get well. Besides, it seemed clear that it was the medical industry that had made me so disabled. I was doing fairly well before I sought medical help.[4]

---

[4] Dr. Richard Deyo made the following observation about the ineffectiveness of various treatments for back pain, and profits as the main reason behind many of these treatments, in an editorial he wrote for

Meanwhile, however, I was in so much pain that I had to keep my children away from me. If they came close, I had to tell them they needed to be very gentle. The worst part was how guilty and responsible for my pain they felt. Sometimes they would ask, "Daddy, did you get hurt lifting us or carrying us?" Having studied child psychology, I knew guilt was a natural childhood response to an unpleasant situation. So I assured them that they were in no way responsible for any of my pain, which I told them had come from driving too much, and that I loved them no matter what.

Also from my studies in psychology, I understood why I would suddenly remember people, places, and events that I had not thought about for years. All these memories signified happier times when I was healthy and free of pain. Remembering such times is one of the strategies the mind employs to deal with unpleasant, painful circumstances. Such defense mechanisms are natural reactions to difficulties like mine.

Every day I prayed and kept up my faith. I knew in my heart that what I was undergoing was all for a good reason, even if I did not know what that reason was. Even if I had to live with pain and disability for the rest of my life, I was grateful for the thirty years of normal life I had had previously. I was determined to do everything I could to learn more and more about this problem so

---

The New England Journal of Medicine: "How can we make true progress in the management of back pain, instead of falling prey to successive fads? . . . Too much research on back problems consists of case series that serve the entrepreneurial purpose of legitimizing expensive new forms of technology, rehabilitation centers, or surgical programs of uncertain effectiveness." Deyo, Richard A., "Fads in the Treatment of Low Back Pain," *The New England Journal of Medicine* 325 (1991), p. 1040. In this editorial he discussed the ineffectiveness of many common treatments for back pain, ranging from steroid and chymopapain injections to lengthy bed rest and traction. Dr. Deyo further stated, "Such fads are not innocuous; they may lead to unnecessary morbidity and costs, as well as to embarrassment for professionals." In other words, some of these ineffective and baseless treatments have actually harmed patients.

that I could keep others from getting into my predicament.

I encouraged my friends and relatives to use good body mechanics and exercise regularly, and I gave them copies of the first good book I read on back care as gifts. In fact, after we bought a NordicTrack cross-country ski machine for my wife, in order to help my friends avoid developing back problems of their own I persuaded three of them to buy these machines too, and I sent others information.

About two and a half months into my stay at home, a quick movement of my eyes brought on a great deal of pain. The muscles in the corners of my eyes hurt. I had a very difficult time reading or focusing. I attributed this new problem to my being home most of the time and not focusing far and near or moving my eyes as much as before. When this problem had persisted for a few days, I went to my family doctor. He found no sign of glaucoma and recommended that I see an ophthalmologist. But I thought I'd better wait. I hoped that after my other problems with pain had been resolved, my eyes would also improve. On top of the eye problems, I had also developed a localized rash, for which my doctor gave me some cortisone ointment. The ointment cleared up the rash, but it would reappear every week or two, and I had to use the medication again. So I had developed another chronic problem.

SHOULDER PAIN

I also began to have pain in my left shoulder. The few stretches and exercises I did for it made it worse; this added a new limitation to my life. I even experienced pain in my ankles and achilles tendon, and a muscle spasm in the bottom of my foot! I remember once, as my therapist was reviewing various stretches and exercises for my back, legs, knees, elbows, shoulder, and foot, we both broke into laughter at the extent of my problems.

Needless to say, my therapist was quite puzzled by all this pain. The best explanation he could give was that shifting my weight around to different parts of my body to avoid pain put too much strain in new areas, and after a while a different muscle or joint began to hurt. As for the sciatica in both my legs, he wondered whether I might have a rare case of herniated disc pressing on both sides of the sciatic nerve. I reminded him that no disc herniation was detected in my spine. At times, however, I was so frustrated by pain and disability that I wished the sciatica was due to a herniated disc so that surgically removing it might at least return my back to normal.

At the same time, I knew from my research and from others who had had surgery that it was not the ultimate cure. My friend who had had his disc removed no longer suffered leg pain, but he still had some back pain and had developed pain in his knees after surgery. He told me that removing a disc can cause a posture imbalance, placing extra pressure on the knees. He had even read in one book that pain in the jaw joints can be due to postural imbalance and can cause back pain. I found this idea hard to believe, but if it were true, I wondered how human beings with such fragile bodies had ever managed to survive for so many thousands of years!

My stomach was still irritated, and the medication was not helping much. While listening to a radio interview I learned about a book called *Foods That Heal,* which describes nutrition-oriented treatments for various illnesses. My wife bought the book. It mentioned a Stanford University study in which cabbage juice had healed all the ulcer patients in the study in less than two weeks, as verified by X-ray.[5] It also mentioned celery as another ulcer healer. Although mine was a case of gastritis, I saw no harm in trying some celery. To my amazement, what medications could not calm, a few sticks of celery did; my stomach was much less irritated after that.

I was also experiencing stomach cramps and a lot of burping, in spite of the fact that I followed a very healthy, low-fat diet, filled with vegetables and fruits. With all these health problems, I felt like an old man. In fact, my mother jokingly said once, "If anyone asks how old you are, just say you're seventy, and they'll

---

[5] Salaman, Maureen, *Foods That Heal* (Menlo Park, Calif.: Statford Publishing, 1989), pp. 458–459. I highly recommend this book.

say, boy, you look so young for your age!" Some mornings I would wake up and wonder, for a moment, whether my recent experiences all had been a dream, a nightmare, and whether I might just get up and walk without pain, somehow miraculously recovered from all this disability. But the moment would pass; I knew recovery could not be that easy.

About this time, my daughter began to have stomach pains. The pain ranged from severe to mild. Her pediatrician ordered a number of tests, the results of which were normal. He wanted to do an upper GI series on her. I asked him to do an ultrasound first. The results of this test were normal too. The pediatrician insisted we should have an upper GI series done, but there was no way I would let my six-year-old daughter be exposed to radiation.

I went to the library and found a book on pediatric illnesses. There it was: recurrent abdominal pain in school-age children. According to *Current Pediatric Diagnosis and Treatment*, more than 90 percent of such cases are due to emotional stress. Usually children between five and ten years old are affected.[6] Obviously, seeing me in pain had taken its toll on my sensitive little girl and caused her abdominal pain. Later on, when I recovered, she also became pain-free. It is inexcusable for a well-trained pediatrician, who has been in practice for many years, not to make the correct diagnosis of a case like this one, when a layman like myself could make the correct diagnosis simply by reading a medical book. If the pediatrician had taken a few minutes to ask some simple questions about my daughter's family life, he would have learned about my condition and realized that since the results of all her tests were normal, the source of her pain must be emotional, not physical.

---

[6] Kemp, C. H. et al., *Current Pediatric Diagnosis and Treatment*, 9th ed. (Norwalk, Conn.: Appleton and Lange, 1987), p. 551.

QUESTIONS AND MORE QUESTIONS

More than three months had passed since I had stayed off work to recover, but there was no significant improvement in my condition. Any small improvement was followed by a setback or pain in another part of my body. I wondered whether I would ever recover completely from this disabling condition. I wondered whether and when I could return to work. My job involved some driving, walking, and standing, and was flexible enough that I was not required to stay in one position for any length of time. But even these minimal job demands had become almost impossible for me to meet. I wondered whether I might have to change my career.

I had always tried to prepare myself mentally and emotionally for permanent injuries resulting from an accident, a disease like cancer, or heart attack or stroke; but I had never imagined that a minor case of back pain could develop to the point of almost total disability. I had been a highly motivated, goal-oriented person; now I could not accomplish anything. If I had become paralyzed in an accident, at least other parts of my body would have been functional and pain-free. Being constantly in pain as I was, however, made practically every activity impossible. In fact, some aspects of various movements had become so restricted due to pain that I could make only what I called "micromovements." At times it appeared to me that I might become so disabled that I would need a wheelchair to get around. I used to smile bitterly at the thought, since I could not sit in a wheelchair long enough for it to be of much use anyway.

I wondered whether I would be able to run again, or sit down comfortably and hold a conversation with a friend. I missed the feeling of walking or working to the point where I became exhausted and my body ached with "good pain." I missed falling asleep because I was tired, not because I was bored. Would I ever be able to sit down on the floor and play with my children again?

Even if my legs, knees, elbows, and other parts of my body recovered from this, I doubted that with two protruded degenerated discs and annular deformity I would ever be able to live an active, normal life again.

I was plagued by questions about my condition that seemed simple, but that my doctors and therapists could not answer.

- Why was it that I did not heal but kept getting worse?
- Weren't all these months of rest and therapy enough?
- Why do so many people in the prime of their lives suffer from back pain? My therapist had told me that most back patients are in their thirties and forties.
- Why are there so many different diagnoses and treatments for back pain?
- Why is it that despite treatments such as surgery many patients experience recurrence of their pain?[7]
- If the pain is due to inflammation, why does taking anti-inflammatory medications not cure the condition? I had taken so much of this medication that I had developed gastritis, but there was no significant improvement in my condition. How much inflammation could I have?

Most of the people I knew with back-related problems were among the nicest people I had ever met. Was back pain the price one had to pay for being nice? One of my coworkers was very athletic, yet he also suffered from recurrent back pain, as well as from sciatica for a time. If weak muscles are the cause of back

---

[7] I knew from my research and from people I knew who had had back surgery that it was not a very effective treatment option; but I was astonished to learn how ineffective surgery for back pain is. According to the Agency for Health Care Policy and Research of United States Department of Health and Human Services, "Surgery has been found to be helpful in only 1 in 100 cases of low back problems. In some people, surgery can even cause more problems. . . . Most back surgery can wait for several weeks without making the condition worse" (U.S. Department of Health and Human Services, Agency for Health Care Policy and Research, *Understanding Acute Low Back Pain Problems*, Publication No. 95-0644 [Rockville, Md., December 1994] p. 12).

pain, why would he experience such symptoms? How strong should back muscles be, anyway? And what about gymnasts and other athletes who put tremendous pressure on their spines; shouldn't they all suffer severe back pain and sciatica? Is there any record of a back-pain epidemic among our ancestors or other cultures in which people rode horses and lived under much harsher conditions? Is back pain the price for the comforts of modern life?

After more than four months of staying home and resting, I had improved in some ways, but had gotten worse in others. My sciatica was somewhat better, but my knees still hurt. I had to place a request for a ramp to be installed over the two steps leading to our apartment. Making this request really made me feel disabled.

I had pain in my elbows, wrists, one shoulder, and eyes, and a chronic rash, to name a few of my health problems. It became obvious to me that staying home much longer might bring about even more pain and disability; I decided it would be better to return to work. So after more than four and half months of staying home, I went back to work. I had lost all my sick leave and vacation time and, on doctor's orders, began working half-time until I could handle working full-time. Every day was a challenge. Every morning I prayed to God Almighty to let me get through the day without a major incident that would require me to stay home again. I still had to avoid sites that involved stairways or walking uphill.

Now I could really appreciate all the modifications made in streets and buildings to accommodate the disabled. The sidewalk ramps at corners made it much easier on my knees to step onto the sidewalk. I also appreciated the long stoplights, which allowed me enough time to cross the street at my own slow pace. Driving was difficult. Pain in my elbows and left shoulder made it hard to steer the car, and looking around when changing lanes or making a turn was quite a task due to pain in my shoulder, eyes, and sensitive neck. I also could not drive faster than forty or so miles an hour; my sciatica kept me from being able to press the gas pedal hard enough to reach higher speeds.

I felt so embarrassed about asking for help that I did whatever necessary to avoid having to, and I had developed various ways of hiding my limitations. If the door to a building or a piece of equipment was too hard to open, I would act as though it was locked so that others would open it for me. I also used to hold something in my right hand or try to find other ways to avoid shaking hands with people.

More than two years had passed since that January morning when I felt my back snap. I had gotten steadily worse, with no prospect of complete recovery. Every day was a struggle, with no end in sight, but I was determined not to give up my search for a cure.

Summary

Now let us take a moment and review the main points discussed so far.

1. As much as 85 percent of back pain cannot be given a definitive diagnosis.
2. A number of scientific studies have revealed that there is no correlation between spinal abnormalities and back pain.
3. It is a myth that herniated disc causes back pain.
4. Conventional treatments for chronic back and neck and hand pain, such as surgery and cortisone shots, have shown very little effectiveness in curing these conditions.
5. Every few years a new treatment for back pain becomes popular among physicians. These treatments often lack scientific proof of their effectiveness and at times cause more harm to patients.
6. The majority of people with back pain are in the prime of their lives, less than fifty years old.
7. Eight out of ten adults and almost four out of ten adolescents suffer from back pain at some point.
8. The treatment of most patients proceeds by trial and error.
9. Most back specialists are puzzled by back pain and are unable to provide plausible explanations for the cause of pain or for its chronicity.
10. All this uncertainty about diagnosis and treatment of back pain has meant months and years of suffering for back-pain patients.
11. **We are in dire need of a correct diagnosis for back pain if we are ever to find a cure!**

3

FINALLY, AN ANSWER

*A*bout a month before I returned to work, we received a flyer in the mail about a book published by Boardroom Classics giving inside information on money, travel, health, and more.[1] By now, experience had taught me how important every bit of information could be in saving time, money, health—even one's life. Since the book offer included a fourteen-day free trial period, I had nothing to lose by ordering the book. It arrived on the day I returned to work.

TENSION MYOSITIS SYNDROME

I began by reading the section on health. Under the topic of back pain, the book mentioned Dr. John Sarno's discovery, as set

---

1 *Bottom Line Personal: The Book of Inside Information* (New York: Boardroom Reports, 1992), pp. 404–405. A number of very useful newsletters are also put out by the same publisher, among them *Bottom Line Health* and *Bottom Line Personal* (Boardroom Reports, Inc., 330 W. 42nd St., New York, NY 10036).

out in his book *Mind over Back Pain*.[2] Dr. Sarno, a professor of clinical rehabilitation medicine at the New York University School of Medicine, discovered that back pain is almost always caused by anger, anxiety, worries, frustration, and tension—not some physical abnormality. He calls this phenomenon tension myositis syndrome (TMS). TMS is the result of reduced blood flow to affected soft tissues. Although extremely painful, the condition is harmless; what is going on is that the subconscious mind is creating pain to distract the person's attention from a stressful relationship or situation.

Once the patient is aware that back pain results from repressed anger and anxiety, the subconscious mind will discontinue its trick, and the pain will stop. TMS sufferers are usually perfectionists who want to be the best in whatever they do and are their own worst critics.

Not Me!

I saw myself as a very calm, positive, easygoing person with a sense of humor, who rarely became angry. Of course, like anyone with chronic back pain I had experienced more pain during or after a stressful period, but was it reasonable to believe that repressed anger and tension could really cause all my pain and disability? And what about my degenerated discs? The medical establishment considers anger and anxiety aggravating factors for existing physical problems, but could tension actually cause these physical problems?

None of my doctors or therapists, nor any of the many books I had read, had yet been able to provide me with a clear explanation, diagnosis, or treatment for back pain and its chronicity. I knew that successful problem solving requires being open-minded and examining all possible solutions.

Considering that this concept of tension myositis syndrome

---

[2] Sarno, John, *Mind over Back Pain* (New York: William Morrow & Company, 1984).

was the observation of a professor of clinical rehabilitation medicine at a major university, I decided to study it further. After all, what could I lose by gaining more knowledge? Even if my pain was not caused by tension, maybe I could help others by learning about it.

MIND OVER BACK PAIN

The local library had a copy of Dr. Sarno's book *Mind over Back Pain*. In this book Dr. Sarno attributed the cause of back pain to reduced blood flow to certain muscle groups as a result of tension. He described back-pain sufferers as conscientious, responsible individuals who are in touch with their feelings (unlike the Type A, aggressive, and competitive personality) and who try to be the best in what they do. They are also their own worst critics. As a result of subconsciously repressing their anger and anxiety, they create a great deal of tension and develop certain physical symptoms, such as back, neck, or shoulder pain. Some individuals even developed sciatica and knee and elbow pain.

Dr. Sarno explained that, unfortunately, the present medical approach to diagnosing back pain is to look only for a structural disorder such as a herniated disc, arthritis, or other physical problems. Such a diagnosis increases the patient's tension level, which causes more pain, and the individual's mobility is restricted by a long list of dos and don'ts that are supposed to prevent further damage to the back.

According to the book, most TMS sufferers are very calm and in control on the conscious level. But their subconscious reacts to repressed anger or tension and causes physical pain. I had always been a fairly calm person who rarely got angry. Even when I did, my anger was usually under control. I wondered how Dr. Sarno's diagnosis could apply to me.

I had also trained myself, since my first course in psychology, to be as free of worry and anxiety as possible. I was taught that people with type A personalities, who get angry easily and are tense, can suffer heart attacks, ulcers, and other ailments. To avoid such ailments, if I could do something about a problem, I would do it. If not, I would be concerned about it and pray about it, but never worry about it or allow it to dominate my thoughts or my life.

When I read about a young girl with chronic back pain who dealt with problems in the same manner I did, though, I became more interested. I also remembered from my course in psychology that one of Freud's patients was a young woman who experienced pain in her right arm. The pain had developed after she failed to write to a loved one before he died. Her subconscious focused the guilt and anger at her right arm, where she experienced pain.

Dr. Sarno gave many examples of patients who had back pain and related problems for years. Many had been diagnosed with structural abnormalities such as herniated disc, and some had had surgery but were never able to recover completely and lead normal, productive lives until they were treated for TMS. These examples gave me the hope that it might be possible for me to lead a normal life again.

Dr. Sarno wrote that reduced blood flow caused the pain. So after I read the book, I lay down, closed my eyes, and imagined an increase in blood flow to my elbows. Strangely enough, the pain in my elbows decreased, but my right triceps muscle began to twitch. It was such a strong twitch that even my wife could see the muscle twitching! This interesting phenomenon indicated to me that what goes on in my mind might affect my painful condition.

But I was not convinced yet. I needed to have a number of questions answered: Do I need to change my personality and show my anger and discontent? How is TMS treated? Are there any doctors in California who diagnose and treat TMS? What is the role of physical therapy and the treatments therapists use to increase blood flow to affected areas? How soon after one realizes that the pain is caused by tension does recovery begin?

HEALING BACK PAIN

After two weeks of calling New York University, I was finally able to talk with Dr. Sarno. He kindly suggested that I read his latest book, *Healing Back Pain*, for answers to my questions. To my amazement, only one copy of this book was to be found in all of the Silicon Valley library system. I placed an immediate request for the book. I also called a bookstore and ordered a copy. Three days later, I checked out the book from the library. I began by reading the appendix, which contained letters from patients who had recovered from chronic back pain simply by reading Dr. Sarno's first book, *Mind over Back Pain*. The success stories contained in those letters—some of whose writers had been in worse condition than I was—gave me more hope for a complete recovery and prepared my mind to be more receptive to the ideas presented in the book. In particular, a letter from a woman who suffered disabling pain similar to mine for seven years and eventually regained complete health represented a clear sign that I could expect the same results.

Therefore, I eagerly began reading the book. Dr. Sarno explained how, in the years since the publication of his first book on tension myositis syndrome in 1984, he had further developed and clarified the concept. In the introduction he mentioned his disappointment with the conventional diagnoses and treatments for chronic back pain. He realized that many of the structural causes blamed for back pain do not actually cause this problem. As he searched for answers, he noticed that 88 percent of back-pain patients suffered or had suffered from other chronic conditions as well. These conditions included the following disorders:

- **Head:** dizziness, ringing in the ears, migraine headaches, sinusitis
- **Cardiopulmonary system:** asthma, allergies, palpitations, high blood pressure
- **Skin:** rashes, acne, hives, psoriasis, warts
- **Gastrointestinal system:** colitis, hiatus hernia, spastic colon, ulcer, irritable bowel syndrome

Since these conditions are caused by repressed anger, anxiety, and tension, Dr. Sarno surmised that chronic back pain might also be caused by tension.

In patients with back pain, tension manifests itself in the postural muscles, nerves, tendons, and ligaments. Its onset is usually attributed to some physical incident, such as lifting a heavy object or being rear ended in a car accident; however, it is minutes, hours, days, or even weeks later before the pain begins, and it is for psychological and emotional reasons that the pain continues for weeks, months, even years. An actual physical injury, such as a broken bone, would heal in a matter of weeks, after which there would be little or no pain.

The Subconscious Mind

Dr. Sarno explained that when TMS sufferers relax or fall asleep, the subconscious mind, where repressed anger and anxiety are stored, induces pain. For that reason, many people feel pain at night or as soon as they have completed their responsibilities and begin to relax. He also mentioned the weekend/vacation syndrome, in which an attack of pain usually occurs during a vacation or on weekends. During these times, when one begins to relax, the buildup of tension is allowed to manifest itself in physical terms. By the end of the vacation or weekend, the person's sense of job responsibility overcomes the pain, and he or she returns to work or other duties.

This phenomenon was exactly what I had experienced. My worst attacks had been on weekends, and usually by Monday I had been able to go to work.[3]

---

[3] I often ask the following question in my seminars: "Have you ever had the experience of being engaged in a long phone conversation or working on the computer for a while, and as soon as the conversation or the work was done, you realized that you had been pressing the phone too hard to your ear or tensing up your neck and shoulders while typing on the computer?" Often, the brain blocks signals from the body and the environment, so that we can focus on the task at

This realization also made me remember that very tense situations, such as when I took one of my incompetent doctors to court, led to severe back pain shortly afterward, whereas other, less tense situations, or thoughts about them, led to pain at a later time. I was perfectly calm on the conscious level but, as the amount of pain indicated, deep inside I was quite angry and upset. The degree of tension affects pain's severity and its onset.

Growing Pains

Dr. Sarno points out that TMS is a cradle-to-grave syndrome. In fact, what we call "growing pains" in children are a manifestation of TMS. Children often have difficulty expressing their feelings and internalize their anger and anxiety, which leads to such pain, especially at night. Both of our children had experienced "growing pains," and we were told by our pediatrician that this experience was very common and nothing to worry about. Indeed, my daughter's recurrent abdominal pain, mentioned earlier, was a case of anxiety-induced pain. Dr. Sarno also mentioned that anyone, at any age, can suffer from TMS, but people who are particularly conscientious are more prone to such symptoms.

None of the many books I had read so far had explained the cause of back pain in such a clear, sensible way. I found myself agreeing more and more with what the doctor had written.

---

hand. That's why it is only after we are done with the task that we begin to notice how hard we were pressing the phone to our ears or how tensed up our muscles had been while we were working on the computer. Even now, you are concentrating on reading this book, and perhaps your mind is blocking signals from your body about how tight your watchband, or your shoes, or your belt feels—except that now you've begun to focus on them!

Conditioning

Reading page 21 of *Healing Back Pain* was the turning point in my long chronic illness. There it was—the heading of the section—Conditioning!

This section explains how we can be conditioned to feel pain not because there is a physical problem with our bodies, but rather because at some point we experienced pain doing certain activities or being in certain positions, and we had come to expect pain during those activities. Dr. Sarno described how at the start of the back pain, an individual may feel pain after sitting for a while; then his or her brain makes the association between sitting and feeling pain in the back. From that point on, whenever the individual sits for a certain period of time, there is a reduction of blood flow to back muscles and the pain begins.

Similarly, because of what people hear from others or are told by the medical establishment, people are conditioned to believe that certain positions or movements put stress on their backs. This belief, of course, programs back-pain patients to expect pain during those activities or in certain positions; therefore, they feel pain. This exact thing had happened to me. I remember a few times when I sneezed at work and was told by my coworkers that sneezing must really hurt. At first it didn't. But after hearing people tell me that it must, I became conditioned to expect pain upon sneezing. Pretty soon every time I sneezed my back hurt too, and I thought my condition was getting worse!

For more than a year I had not been able to sit comfortably longer than twenty minutes at a time, and even at that I need to sit on a four-inch foam cushion. My right piriformis muscle was so sensitive that if I ignored this time limit, the muscle would go into spasm and initiate sciatica in my right leg. And sometimes if I ignored this time limit and sat longer, my back began to hurt.

In my first year of college psychology I had learned that we are conditioned from childhood to feel and behave in certain ways, and that by using what are called behavior modification techniques we can gradually change those conditioned responses into whatever we want. Using those techniques, I had been able to act as my own psychotherapist and trainer and gradually overcome many of my fears (such as my fear of public speaking) and begin new habits (such as regular exercise).

I also knew that a conditioned response can lose its intensity and eventually be eliminated if no reward is given. Physiologist Ivan Pavlov used to ring a bell each time he fed a group of dogs. After repeating this procedure a few times, the dogs automatically salivated each time the bell rang, even when no food was provided.[4] However, in such a case, if the bell is rung continuously and no food (reward) is provided, the dogs eventually stop salivating.

Thus, as soon as I realized that my body had been conditioned to feel pain when I sat down for more than twenty minutes, I continued to sit as I read on with no worry that I was doing myself physical harm. By ignoring the pain, I deprived my subconscious of the reward it wanted; when it became convinced I would no longer give it the reward of my attention, it would eventually stop causing pain.

THE PSYCHOLOGY OF TMS

Dr. Sarno explained how by repressing our unkind, childish, selfish, and other unacceptable feelings in the face of circumstances that involve pleasing others, the subconscious mind protects us from facing such unacceptable emotions. It diverts our

---

[4] Our bodies are also conditioned to respond to environmental stimulus. When we see a police car with red flashing lights in our car's rearview mirror, our bodies respond by increasing our heart rates. Some people feel sudden pangs of hunger when they notice it's lunchtime, when a few moments earlier they were not hungry. How about those times when you are too tired to move another muscle, and the phone rings? Have you noticed how suddenly you find the energy to get up and answer the telephone? These are some examples of conditioned responses in people.

attention by causing some physical disorder. This diversion is part of what psychoanalysts call a defense mechanism.

For example, if you have an elderly mother who is ill, the demands her illness place on you can create an emotional conflict. On the one hand, you know that the right thing to do is to take care of her; on the other hand, taking care of her disrupts your life and makes it difficult to meet your own needs. As a conscientious son or daughter, you do the right thing and consider your own needs unacceptable and selfish. But if your anger and resentment about the situation are great enough, and your mother is very demanding, you could experience back pain. Also, first-time parents who have to deal with the demands of caring for a newborn may experience a similar situation and develop back pain.

For another example, imagine that your supervisor at work has a habit of humiliating you in front of everyone. You might be calm about it and cope very well on the surface. You might tell yourself, *That's just how she is,* or *It's not worth getting upset about.* However, at a deep level you might experience anger, frustration, helplessness, and other negative feelings, which when repressed can lead to such physical disorders as back pain. [5]

Sometimes people with chronic pain tell me that there are no serious problems facing them that can account for so much pain. The fact is that the source of anger, anxiety, and frustration does not have to be some serious problem. As the following case illustrates, the source of anger can be something as simple as a dripping faucet.

One of my friends had a roommate who never shut off a par-

---

[5] In addition, most of us have been led to believe that our backs are weak and fragile. Any incident that causes the slightest pain or discomfort can cause great deal of worry and anxiety and lead to TMS. That sequence of events is why many people report waking up to back pain or numbness in their legs or arms days or weeks after such an incident. One of my friends, who was diagnosed with a herniated disc and was able to avoid surgery by learning the information presented in this book, told me that his back pain began because he was worrying about some heavy lifting he did at work.

ticular faucet completely, so the faucet dripped constantly. My friend did not like to waste water. He talked to his roommate about the problem, but since they did not get along, the roommate began to let not only that particular faucet drip, but all the other faucets in the apartment as well. This behavior created so much anger and frustration for my friend that soon after he began to have back pain.

Of course, these feelings are much more intense when parents, spouses, children, and loved ones cause your anger and anxiety. In rare cases, anger might be due to a very traumatic experience in childhood, and feelings of anger and anxiety are repressed to such an extent that a person is completely unaware of them on the conscious level. However, in a majority of cases people are aware that the pain is due to personal conflicts or other stressful situations.[6]

I was quite familiar with various manifestations of the de-

---

[6] This concept might be unfamiliar to some; however, our emotions constantly lead to physiological changes. When we feel embarrassed, the blood vessels just beneath the skin on our faces dilate, making us blush. When we are frightened, the same blood vessels constrict, and our faces turn pale. We get goose bumps when excited, and dry mouths or sweaty palms when nervous. Even thoughts can produce physiological changes. When we think about a lemon or imagine several times biting into one, most of us begin to salivate. What physical changes, then, might be produced by repeated thoughts about other ideas or words, especially emotionally loaded words like *divorce,* and stressful life situations, such as a job interview? Norman Cousins of UCLA Medical School explains in detail many cases and studies dealing with positive and negative emotions and their effects on the body. *Head First: The Biology of Hope* (New York: Dutton, 1989) is the result of years of research and observation of this phenomenon. In fact, due to the extensive research being conducted in this field, *Consumer Reports* published an encyclopedic book to which more than thirty physicians and researchers contributed. The book is titled *Mind/Body Medicine: How to Use Your Mind for Better Health* (Yonkers, N.Y.: Consumer Reports Books, 1993) and features the works of researchers from Harvard and Duke to Yale and Stanford Universities.

fense mechanisms the mind employs in order to avoid dealing with unpleasant thoughts and situations. But the defense mechanisms I knew about were all related to various mental and emotional states. One such defense mechanism is denial.

When a person faces an event or circumstance that he or she finds unacceptable—such as the sudden loss of a loved one, a diagnosis of cancer, or drug abuse by a family member—denial protects the person from the immediate shock of facing the devastating news and allows for gradual absorption of reality. Another defense mechanism is regression. One aspect of regression is that the person, when faced with unpleasant and unacceptable circumstances, remembers earlier, happier times. I had experienced this phenomenon during my painful ordeal when places, people, and events that signified happier, healthier periods in my life suddenly came to mind.

That a physical disorder could serve as another defense mechanism sounded reasonable to me. In his book Dr. Sarno listed a number of TMS equivalents that also serve as defense mechanisms. These include pre-ulcer states, various gastrointestinal illnesses, high blood pressure, hay fever and asthma, headaches, acne, eczema, warts and other skin disorders, dizziness, frequent urination, and even heart palpitations.[7]

At the end of the chapter on the psychology of TMS, Dr. Sarno presented the good news that overcoming TMS does not require a personality change. Simply knowing that the pain is due to negative emotions and changing one's perception about the source of one's pain can do wonders in the treatment of TMS.

---

[7] As mentioned in the introduction, prior to his discovery of TMS, Dr. Sarno noticed that 88 percent of his patients had histories of one or more of these disorders, all of which appeared likely to be tension-related. This observation was what led him to the logical conclusion that since the primary tissues involved in back pain were muscles of the neck, shoulder, back, and buttocks, tension might also be the cause of this condition.

THE PHYSIOLOGY OF TMS

Dr. Sarno explained that the autonomic nervous system is responsible for these physical changes. The autonomic nervous system controls blood flow to various parts of the body, rate of breathing, heart rate, body temperature, release of gastric juices in the stomach, and other bodily functions that occur automatically, with no need for us to regulate or think about them. Any of these functions can be affected in response to repressed anger and tension, especially at night when the conscious mind is asleep and the subconscious is not restrained. For this reason, many people experience pain at night or when they wake up. Now I understood why I woke up to sciatica and abdominal pain and why my hands went numb at night.[8]

Finally I could see clearly why for the past two years I had experienced TMS in my back and TMS equivalents such as rash, shortness of breath, gastritis, and stomach cramps, to name a few. I understood how being raised in a family where the parents constantly argued and fought had affected my health. For the past seventeen years I had suffered from hay fever and acne. I was also told during a medical exam that I have heart palpitations, which is a harmless but common condition. I had noticed for the past several years that when I ignored the acne on my face, it cleared up. My hay fever had been seasonal, but one particular year, it turned into asthma attacks, especially at night. Of course, now I know why. That year I had been in a serious car accident and in a very stressful situation that had caused me a great deal of resentment and anger.

I also recognized how my back pain had begun and continued due to marital conflicts. The problems at home coupled with a tense 100-mile-a-day commute had left me little opportunity to rest and relax, both physically and mentally. My experiences with back specialists and therapists had added to my anger and frustrations, and had led to more pain. My wife, too, had suffered her

---

[8] In my experience, the timing of pain is one of the best indicators of whether the pain is TMS-related or not.

share of back pain, headaches, and high blood pressure; she was diagnosed with scoliosis (curvature of the spine), osteoarthritis, and degenerated discs as causes of her back pain.

It became clear to me that at some point in my life I had developed these bodily responses to tension, and later they had become conditioned responses—habits. It was certainly time to change these bad habits![9]

By this time I had sat reading Dr. Sarno's book for about an hour and a half. My piriformis muscle was not hurting much anymore, but my lower back, especially my tailbone, was killing me. If I had not just learned about TMS, I probably would have lay down and used ice to ease the pain. As this pain could not make me get up, it shifted to my right knee, and later to the front of my neck, where I had never experienced pain before. It became clear to me that as real as the pain felt, it was indeed a trick that my subconscious was playing on me. It was reducing blood flow to my back, knee, and neck to cause pain in order to keep me occupied with physical symptoms.

This phenomenon is not strange to those with chronic pain. In fact, they are quite familiar with pain moving from one part of their bodies to another. This phenomenon used to cause me a great deal of worry, as I believed it meant that my condition was getting worse. However, now that I knew the pain was due to reduction of blood flow, movement of pain from one part of my body to another was no longer a source of worry and anxiety.

I remembered one of the letters Dr. Sarno included in his book, in which a back patient described a similar experience. The man had been diagnosed as having a herniated disc pressing on the right side of his sciatic nerve, giving him right-leg pain; but

---

[9] During the time when I experienced shortness of breath, if my family doctor, instead of reassuring me that this was due to stress, had told me that since I suffer from hay fever this could be an allergy attack or asthma, prescribed tests, and given me medications, shortness of breath could have become a conditioned response too, and I could have become asthmatic. Caring, conscientious doctors can indeed make a world of difference in their patients' lives.

when he learned about TMS, his left leg began to hurt also. He had never had a problem before with his left leg, and when the left-leg pain began, he laughed with joy, realizing that his pain was not due to a herniated disc.

THE TREATMENT OF TMS

Dr. Sarno explained that "The treatment rests on two pillars: (1) the acquisition of knowledge, of insight into the nature of the disorder, and (2) the ability to act on the knowledge and thereby change the brain's behavior."[10]

When the patient realizes that the pain is simply a manifestation of repressed anger and anxiety, he or she takes the first step toward recovery. Dr. Sarno highly recommends talking to the brain (the subconscious mind), and even getting mad at it for causing so much pain. This technique may seem silly to those not familiar with psychology or the subconscious mind, but it is extremely effective.

In fact, we all have experienced talking to ourselves in order to take conscious control of certain physiological responses caused by our emotions. Most of us have experienced being sad enough to feel like crying while in public. However, as tears come to our eyes, we decide that this is not the time or the place to cry. By telling ourselves not to cry or simply deciding to stop the tears, we consciously stop the process. The same is true for laughter or itching. This innate ability we all possess can also help us eliminate back pain.

Researchers at the University of California at Davis discovered that patients who received detailed information about their operation prior to surgery and told themselves not to bleed from the part of body being operated on reduced blood loss by as much as 50 percent![11] Thus, you can have a significant impact on your

---

[10] John E. Sarno, M.D., *Healing Back Pain* (New York: Warner Books, 1991), p. 77.
[11] Goleman, Daniel and Joel Gurin, *Mind-Body Medicine* (Yonkers, N.Y.: Consumer Reports Books, 1993), pp. 410–411. Robert Baker,

body's physiological responses simply by talking to it.[12]

Dr. Sarno also recommends physical activity, especially rigorous activity, to overcome fears of bending, walking, lifting, and so on; and he suggests discontinuing all physical treatment. Until the patient renounces all physical treatment, from physical therapy to acupuncture, he or she is still hanging on to the belief that some structural problem is to blame. Focusing on that possibility causes the pain and other symptoms to continue.[13]

New students of Dr. Sarno's methods commonly ask how soon after conscious acceptance of the diagnosis one may become pain-free. Dr. Sarno points out that the subconscious mind is slow

---

M.D., *Successful Surgery: A Doctor's Mind-Body Guide to Help You Through Surgery* (New York: Pocket Books, 1996).

[12] Dr. Sarno pointed out that there is much we do not understand about the workings of the brain; however, the fact that since 1973 he has successfully treated thousands of back patients is sufficient proof that his method of talking to the brain and reminding oneself daily that TMS is a harmless condition works. We constantly talk to ourselves anyway. When things go wrong, such as being late for an appointment, we say things such as, *I should have left earlier,* or *I should not have taken the freeway.* There are many occasions when we talk to ourselves and give ourselves positive or negative messages. So why not send our minds the necessary messages to stop the pain? Psychologist and best-selling author Dr. Shad Helmstetter has written a number of books on the power and effectiveness of positive self-talk. In *The Self-Talk Solution* (New York: William Morrow, 1987), he discussed in detail the relationship between the subconscious mind and self-talk, and the great results positive self-talk can produce. Keep in mind, too, that it is not just the workings of the brain that are yet to be fully understood; our knowledge concerning the mechanism of action of many medications is limited as well.

[13] Of course, if one believes that these treatments help, or physical therapy and other physical treatments provide some relief from tension, they can bring about temporary relief. At the beginning, physical therapy was very helpful to me. The first therapist was very helpful and confident, but later, when different therapists took care of me and I found the visits frustrating, the therapy became a source of tension and made my condition worse.

to change. Reminding oneself once a day that TMS and not some structural disorder is the reason for the pain can bring about significant pain reduction within two to six weeks, and eventual recovery afterward.

Now I began to realize why physical therapy at times made my condition worse. By focusing on the part of the body that was in pain—stretching and exercising it—I actually reinforced the mind-caused pain and created more pain. If I had ignored the pain, as I did for the first nine months, it would have remained insignificant due to my indifference to it.[14]

I knew from my past experience with the subconscious mind that it essentially acts like a preschooler, and as I will explain later, treating it as such can facilitate recovery and help in controlling other TMS equivalents as well. As with a typical preschooler, if you ignore bad behavior and keep repeating the same commands, as Dr. Sarno suggests, sooner or later the subconscious realizes that it can no longer attract any attention and will give up misbehaving. Of course, it will give up much faster if there is a reward for good behavior, as will be demonstrated in the story of my own recovery.

Dr. Sarno also discussed the results of a follow-up survey of his patients. That survey, conducted in 1987, tracked a group of patients whose diagnosis of herniated disc had

---

[14] The validity of Dr. Sarno's advice to ignore the pain was demonstrated in the following study conducted in Finland and published in *The New England Journal of Medicine*. Three groups of patients with acute, nonspecific low back pain were compared for their speed of recovery. "The patients were randomly assigned to one of three treatments: bed rest for two days (67 patients), back-mobilization exercises (52 patients), or the continuation of ordinary activities as tolerated (the control group; 67 patients). . . . After three and twelve weeks, the patients in the control group had better recovery than those prescribed bed rest or exercise." Researchers concluded, "Among patients with acute low back pain, continuing ordinary activities within the limits permitted by the pain leads to more rapid recovery than either bed rest or back mobilization exercises." Malmivaara, Antti, et al, *The New England Journal of Medicine* 332 (1995): 351–355.

been documented by CT scan and who had been through Dr. Sarno's TMS program between 1983 and 1986. Dr. Sarno's treatment was successful for 88 percent (ninety-six patients); 10 percent (eleven patients) had improved, but continued to experience some pain and restricted activity; and only 2 percent (two patients) experienced no change. The two patients whose conditions did not improve suffered from severe, persistent psychological problems.

Despite such great results, Dr. Sarno has found the medical establishment resistant to accepting the TMS diagnosis. Some of his critics say that tension might be the cause of pain for 30 to 40 percent of the patients, but not the majority. Dr. Sarno wonders why these critics never make the TMS diagnosis for their patients. I certainly had seen firsthand how back specialists are only concerned with physical aspects of back pain and have little interest in their patients as people. The TMS diagnosis would require these specialists to get to know their patients in order to determine the source of tension in their lives. Back specialists would have to spend more than a few minutes with each patient, which, among other drawbacks, would not be cost-effective!

Besides the survey just described, Dr. Sarno pointed out in his book that in most people the discs in the neck and low back, because of activity in those locations, wear out by the age of twenty, but the result is not pain. Millions of people with degenerated discs never have back pain. So my degenerated discs are perfectly normal. This information helped to remove any worries I had, consciously and subconsciously, about a structural problem with my spine and further damage to it.[15]

---

[15] Many studies on people without back pain have shown no relation between spinal abnormalities and back pain. As mentioned in the introduction a recent study, which received national attention, used magnetic resonance imaging (MRI) to demonstrate the presence of bulging, degenerated, and herniated discs in majority of the subjects, as well as spondylolysis and other abnormalities. This study casts serious doubts on the current method of diagnosis and treatment of back pain, and proves that most spinal abnormalities do not cause back

Age and TMS

Dr. Sarno also pointed out that the majority of back-pain sufferers are in their thirties, forties, and fifties, and fewer are in their sixties and seventies. If back pain were due to some degenerative process, the largest group suffering from it would be the elderly. The responsibilities and pressures that the younger group face are the real reasons for their pain. This information helped me understand why the majority of back patients I met in physical therapy were in their thirties and forties.[16]

CONVENTIONAL DIAGNOSES AND TREATMENTS

Dr. Sarno explained how diagnoses given for back pain—ranging from inflammation and herniated disc to scoliosis, fiberomyalgia, and osteoarthritis—are rarely responsible for the pain. Conventional treatments serve mainly as placebos; they are effective for a while, but the patient begins to experience recurrence of the pain or some other TMS equivalent later, due to tension. For this reason, surgery does not eliminate the pain in most cases.

Once I met a man in his forties who had developed pain in various parts of his body over a ten-year period. Every time he

---

pain. The editorial on this study also mentioned that up to 85 percent of back patients cannot be given a definitive diagnosis for their pain (Maureen C. Jensen, et al., "Magnetic Resonance Imaging of the Lumbar Spine in People Without Back Pain," *The New England Journal of Medicine* 331 (July 14, 1994): 69–73.) Many earlier studies, listed in the introduction, have also confirmed this finding.

[16] According to the survey presented in *Backache Relief*, the majority of back patients are less than forty-five years old (p. 200); 72 percent are between the ages of nineteen and forty-nine, and 44 percent are between the ages of thirty and forty-nine (p. x). Also, as mentioned in the introduction, 36 percent of adolescents suffer from back pain by the age of fifteen.

sought medical help, he ended up with surgery. He was operated on for back pain, knee pain, neck pain, hand pain, and was still suffering from chronic pain. I really felt sorry for him.

Other conventional diagnoses for chronic pain in other parts of body caused by tension include:

- Chondromalacia patella (roughening of knee caps)
- Bone spurs
- Plantar fasciitis
- Neuroma (foot and heel pain)
- Tendinitis (tennis elbow)
- Bursitis

Temporamandibular joint syndrome (TMJ) refers to pain in the jaw joints. I had received several diagnoses and treatments for this condition and used to suffer from it frequently prior to my back pain. Now I realized that my jaw pain was the result of my not speaking up about issues that angered me.

One of the amazing things about back-pain treatment is the number of practitioners in this field. I remember reading in *Backache Relief* that often a patient would be treated by many different doctors and specialists and improve only a little or get worse, but after a visit or two to the chiropractor or acupuncturist, the patient's back pain would disappear. And of course there are those who became worse from going to a chiropractor and got better after seeing a doctor.

Now I understood the reason for these disparate outcomes: the real factor in most treatments for the back is the patient's state of mind. If the patient trusts the practitioner and believes what is said, and above all feels confident about the treatment's effectiveness, he or she will improve or recover. For a physical problem such as a broken bone to heal, the patient does not have to believe in or get along with the doctor. Although the patient's attitude and emotional state can affect recovery, we do not see, for example, an epidemic of broken bones that do not heal among young people.

The same kind of dynamic can be at work even when you are reading a book. The first book I read carefully on back pain and proper body mechanics was very well written, with exact figures on how each position reduces pressure to the spine in square inches. I felt very confident about the usefulness of the information provided in the book and experienced little or no pain as long as I followed its instructions. Of course, if while receiving a certain treatment a patient experiences a decrease in the stress and tension in his or her life—for example, if the patient's job situation improves—this also helps the recovery. In such cases, however, most patients associate their recovery with the treatment rather than reduction or elimination of their tension.

Another good illustration that back pain is a mental phenomenon is my experience of helping people recover from back pain over the phone. They begin to improve as I tell them about my experiences and rapid recovery. Relating my experience with recovery creates so much positive emotion and excitement that people get better while I am talking to them. This demonstrates once again that a positive change in a patient's emotional state and increase in knowledge can bring about rapid improvements and recovery. Such a happy outcome is impossible for an actual physical injury, such as a broken bone.

I am often asked in my seminars about chiropractic treatment. In the case of chiropractic treatment, besides the mental factor, we are also dealing with a reflex response. In the same way that your hand automatically pulls back when you touch something hot in order to prevent a serious burn, a chiropractor's work on your back can act as a reflex response, sending a signal to your brain to reduce pain. The problem is that—like all other physical treatments, which act as placebos—chiropractic treatment brings about only temporary relief, and most patients require adjustments several times a week or month.

MIND AND BODY

In the last chapter of his book, Dr. Sarno discussed at some length the mind/body connection and studies demonstrating how emotions affect various bodily functions and organs. He cited a number of studies to illustrate this point, among them Dr. Dean Ornish's landmark study on the effects of positive emotions as a part of a healthy lifestyle to reverse heart disease.[17]

Dr. Sarno also discussed in more detail the mental aspects of TMS and TMS equivalents. He pointed out that it is not essential for us to know how the mind causes these symptoms; what matters is that being aware of their origin causes the mind to stop the pain and allows us to lead a normal life.[18]

FREQUENTLY ASKED QUESTIONS

These are some of the questions individuals and audiences frequently ask me:

Q: *Are you saying that all back pain is caused by tension?*

A: No! A variety of disorders and diseases, such as cancer, bone disease, and infections, can cause back pain. The Agency for Health Care Policy and Research of the U.S. Department of Health and Human Services concluded that one in two hundred cases of back pain is due to a serious disorder—that's one-half of 1 percent. Even though the likelihood of a serious physical disorder is slight, it is imperative to be examined by a physician, especially for your first episode of back pain.

You can also experience back pain due to an actual injury. My brother-in-law has a black belt in tae kwon do and is very flexible and well built. However, once while moving a refrigerator he twisted his back. He felt pain in his back immediately, and for

---

[17] This book, *Dr. Ornish's Program for Reversing Heart Disease* (New York: Random House, 1990), provides another excellent testament to the fact that our emotions indeed affect our health. Interestingly enough, Dr. Ornish also discussed how, as part of a comprehensive program, the patients used self-talk to open up blocked arteries.

[18] The explanation of TMS provided here has been sufficient for those I have worked with to understand the relationship between tension and pain and recover. You may wish to consult Dr. Sarno's *Healing Back Pain* for a more in-depth understanding of TMS.

a few days could not move from the pain. However, he gradually improved, and after three weeks he had completely recovered. As in this example, when an injury is physical, it will eventually heal. However, if you continue to have pain for weeks and months, then you should consider tension and/or conditioning as a possible cause of your pain.

Q: *So how do I know whether my back pain is due to an injury or is from tension?*

A: If any of the following conditions exist, you probably have TMS:

1. The pain persists or recurs or both, despite rest and various treatments.
2. The pain has no clear cause or can be attributed only to a physical incident that happened a while back, such as lifting an object two weeks earlier.
3. The pain is attributed to a routine activity, such as driving, sitting too long, mowing the lawn, or playing golf.
4. The pain pattern matches TMS: You hurt or have more pain at night, first thing in the morning, or on weekends. The pain moves around from your back to your leg or your shoulder. You should also watch for pain that comes long after an activity or at the end of the workday.[19]
5. The pain is sharp, not the dull muscle ache you get from too much work or exercise.

---

[19] A test engineer friend of mine, who had recovered rapidly from whiplash, was experiencing pain and numbness in his hands. He was worried about having carpal tunnel syndrome (CTS). When I told him CTS is another manifestation of tension, he was very skeptical. He blamed working on the computer as the cause of pain. I knew it was from trying to complete his master's degree while working full-time and raising three children. One day as he was driving home from work, his hands hurt so bad that he drove directly to the doctor's office. However, this incident made him realize that the pain was related to tension, he applied my techniques and recovered.

6. Numbness is intermittent. It gets better or worse and moves around.
7. There is no change in color or swelling in the "injured" area. Our bodies are made to respond immediately to a serious injury. Can you see an actual swelling or change in color in the injured area? If not, the pain could very well be TMS.

Since my recovery I have been injured several times while sparring in my karate class or in other incidents, and I have found that two or three days of rest is about what I need to recover from the initial injury. After that I test my ability to walk or work and push back against the pain until I have recovered completely. I remember once, two weeks after I had recovered from being kicked in the arms repeatedly during sparring, I woke one night in pain. I could not determine why, but I knew it had to be due to either tension or conditioning. I quickly eliminated the pain and went back to sleep.

Q: *How do I know the pain is in my head?*

A: I am asked this question quite often. People think that a diagnosis of TMS implies that the pain is in their heads and is not real. As explained earlier, pain and numbness are caused by reduction of blood flow to the affected muscles and nerves. So there is a real physiological change in your body that causes the pain; for this reason, warming or cooling the area helps increase the blood flow and reduce the pain. In the same way that, when you are under severe stress, your face may turn pale (due to a reduction of blood flow to your face), your mouth may become dry, or your palms feel cold and sweaty, a real physiological change causes the pain.

Q: *How do I know my back pain is not from too much work?*

A: You will know if your pain is from too much work when the pain is what I call a "good pain." You feel tired and somewhat relaxed; most important, the pain subsides after a day or two with some rest or with more exercise or more work.

Q: *What role do chiropractors play?*
A: Chiropractic treatments provide temporary relief due to the placebo effect and the reflex response. As with all other physical treatments for this condition, the patient's belief that chiropractic treatment will reduce pain will lead to an actual reduction of pain. In addition to the placebo effect, the chiropractor's manipulation of the back can act as a reflex response, sending a message to the brain to reduce pain immediately. However, as with all other treatments that do not deal with the actual cause of chronic back pain, relief is only temporary, and one needs additional treatments.

Q: *What about the placebo effect?*
A: All physical treatments for TMS-related back pain are simply placebos. They work because patients believe they bring some relief. Studies mentioned earlier have shown that these treatments do not cure chronic back, neck, or hand pain. For the few who find permanent relief through physical treatments—such as surgery, cortisone shots, and chiropractic manipulation—other tension-related ailments, such as high blood pressure, ulcers, and headaches, may subsequently emerge in place of the back pain.

Alternatively, the treatment may be successful only because it coincided with a positive change in life circumstances that created tension. This positive change in back pain sufferers' emotional situation leads to the elimination of pain, which they naturally attribute to the treatment. In contrast, treating TMS gets to the root of the problem, and for most people leads to complete recovery with no need for repeated treatments.

Q: *What about meditation and relaxation techniques?*
A: Although meditation and relaxation techniques have many health benefits and are very useful, by themselves they too act as placebos and bring only temporary relief. The first step in recov-

ering from TMS is realizing that the pain is tension-related. Once you recognize this fact and begin to deal with the root of the problem, then meditation and relaxation can be quite helpful for faster recovery.

Q: *What about misalignment of the spine?*
A: This theory is another big myth. What evidence is there to show that our backs go out of alignment every few weeks or months and need adjustments?

TMS EQUIVALENTS

The following are other physical manifestations of tension that I have observed.

1. Spasms: When a person is agitated about something and, consciously or unconsciously, represses those thoughts and feelings, they can manifest themselves as muscle spasms in various parts of the body. Spasm is the involuntary, often powerful, contraction of muscles.

a. Bronchial asthma: This is a condition of the lung characterized by widespread narrowing of the airways due to spasm of the smooth muscles.[20] A professor who suffered from seven years of chronic bronchitis recovered rapidly following the techniques discussed in the upcoming chapters.

b. Angina: One of the causes of angina is spasm of coronary arteries, in which blood vessels narrow suddenly for a short time, leading to reduction of blood flow and chest pain.[21]

c. Hiccups: The diaphragm helps us breathe. However, when it goes into spasm, we experience hiccups.[22]

---

[20] *Stedman's Medical Dictionary* (New York: Houghton Mifflin, 1995).
[21] American Medical Association Encyclopaedia of Medicine (New York: Random House, 1989).
[22] A hazardous materials specialist, who had attended my seminar and

d. **Leg cramps:** These usually happen at night and are another manifestation of tension.

e. **Spastic colon:** The name says it all.

f. **Facial tics:** These are caused by spasm of the facial muscles.

2. **Teeth grinding:** This physical manifestation of repressed rage and agitation happens during sleep. An executive assistant who had attended my rapid recovery seminar told me that the recovery plan helped her not only to eliminate her neck and shoulder pain, but also to stop grinding her teeth at night. She had been prescribed a mouth guard to wear at night to protect her teeth.

3. **Most acquired allergies:** When an allergy is acquired, an individual who previously did not have an allergic reaction to a certain substance suddenly develops asthma, hay fever, a rash, or other allergic symptoms. I have found that most people who recover from TMS also recover from such allergic reactions as well.

4. **Warts:** This and most other skin conditions are caused by tension. As you may recall, in researching the cause of my sudden episode of rash, I learned that the causes of most skin conditions are not known.

5. **Sensitive teeth:** If you suffer from a chronic case of sensitive teeth, this might be your body's way of manifesting tension.

6. **Canker sores:** This and a number of other chronic mouth- and teeth-related conditions can be caused by tension.

7. **Calcium deposits:** A friend of mine recovered rapidly from chronic pain in his right heel that had been diagnosed as calcium deposits and avoided surgery.

---

recovered from chronic back pain within 48 hours, told me that she suffered from chronic hiccups for a long time. On the advice of a friend, she went to a quiet place and focused her mind to stop them, and it worked. She also told me that using my techniques helped her recover from recurrent tendinitis in her arm.

8. Hereditary hemorrhagic telangiectasia: This hereditary condition is characterized by bleeding from red spots that could be in the nose, lungs, brain, or other parts of the body. It manifests itself after puberty and in some cases can be fatal. I will discuss in detail one such case that was treated successfully using the rapid recovery plan.

The graphic on the next page summarizes the causes of back and neck pain. It is further explained on the following page.

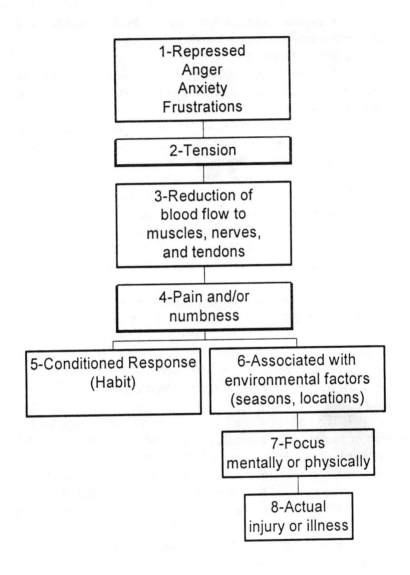

1. Repressed anger, anxiety, worries, frustrations, and a host of negative emotions create tension.

2. Same as number 1.

3. Tension causes a reduction of blood flow to various muscles, nerves, ligaments, and tendons in the back, neck, shoulder, legs, arms, knees, and so on.

4. This reduction of blood flow to the muscles, nerves, ligaments, and tendons can cause pain and numbness (pain might be attributed to a physical incident, or begin with no apparent cause).

5. Regardless of how the pain began, it becomes a conditioned response—a habit—and thus becomes chronic. Thus, when you get into certain positions or perform certain movements, there is a reduction of blood flow to your muscles and nerves which causes pain or numbness. Keep in mind that as severe as the pain feels, it is harmless and by no means related to some structural disorder.

6. Your pain may also be triggered due to a conditioned response associated with changes in the environment, such as cold weather, or locations, such as your place of employment. In severe cases, if a particular person is the source of your tension, the scent of their cologne or perfume, even in their absence, can act as a trigger for your brain to reduce blood to your back and cause pain!

7. The body part you focus on mentally can become the target of tension. If you constantly worry about injuring your back or hand, or you believe you are in a high-risk group for injuring yourself, it is very likely that you will get back pain or hand pain. Also, the part of the body you focus on physically can experience pain. Sometimes when tension builds up and you no longer want to do any more than you have to, you may feel pain in a part of your body that prevents you from taking on more work or responsibility. I have seen cases of back pain, leg pain, bronchitis, carpal tunnel syndrome, rash, and so on that have protected people from taking on more work or more responsibility—forcing them to take a vacation! [23]

---

[23] Philosophically speaking, if we cannot stand it any longer, our

8. An actual physical injury can become chronic due to tension and conditioning. All the worries and anxieties related to an injury can create enough tension that the pain and disability will persist despite the healing of the original injury.

The best indicator of a tension-related condition is that the pain manifests itself usually when you complete a task and begin to relax, such as at the end of a workday, on a weekend, or during a vacation. It can also manifest itself at night, during sleep, or when you wake up in the morning.

Now that you know the diagnosis, let's begin the recovery process.

---

backs hurt, and we lie down. If we feel we cannot go on any more, our legs or knees begin to hurt. If it is too much to handle, we experience pain in our arms and hands. When we carry too much burden, our shoulders hurt. And if we want to talk back and we do not or cannot, our jaws feel the pain!

4

RAPID RECOVERY

*N*ow I had to combine my newly gained knowledge of TMS, my experiences with behavior modification techniques and conditioning, and years of experience with my subconscious, to overcome back pain, sciatica in both legs, knee pain, elbow pain, shoulder pain, a sensitive neck, eczema, gastritis, stomach cramps, and other health problems.

I reread the chapter on treatment of TMS in order to fully understand Dr. Sarno's approach. He suggests that patients should resume physical activity as soon as they feel confident about the diagnosis and experience a significant reduction in pain. He warns that becoming too active prematurely may induce pain and frighten the person, retarding recovery. He recommends a slow but consistent progress, which helps build the patient's confidence in the diagnosis and takes about two to six weeks to work.

I had lived with this pain for more than twenty-five months. That's twenty-five months of not carrying my children, not being a whole person, and constantly saying, "I can't, I can't, I can't." Now that I had found the answers to my questions, it was too difficult to wait two to six weeks to get better. I wanted to get well and live a full life right away. I also wanted to have a better way of measuring progress and building my confidence, rather than just wait for recovery to happen.

With these thoughts going through my mind, I continued to study the section on Dr. Sarno's treatment program. He mentioned the case of an attorney in his mid-thirties who had become pain-free within weeks of going through the program. But the attorney was still afraid to run, though he could do other activities more strenuous than running. So, after a year, when he ran, the pain returned. He continued running, however, and a few nights later, when he woke up with upper back pain, he realized that it was TMS. After that, he was all right.

So fear of pain is the key reason for limits on one's activities. But in the face of determination and a strong will, fear does not stand a chance. The level of fear is one reason why some patients recover almost immediately after learning about TMS, whereas others take days or weeks. In his book Dr. Sarno mentioned a letter from a patient who had been diagnosed with a herniated disc as the cause of his back pain, with surgery recommended as treatment. Upon reading *Mind over Back Pain,* he decided to ignore his severe back pain and went for a four-hour drive, after which he was free of pain.

DESIGNING MY RECOVERY PLAN

The thought of immediate recovery was very exciting to me. Considering the extent of my pain and disability, though, I deemed it unwise to simply get up and go.

I usually try to take a calm, methodical approach to solving problems and reaching my goals. I had been quite successful in the past in meeting a number of personal and career challenges by doing so. Thus, I decided to design a step-by-step recovery plan that would ensure a safe yet rapid recovery from more than twenty-five months of pain.[1] In designing the plan I had to consider the following:

---

[1] At this point in my seminars I usually ask, "Since back pain is caused by repressed negative emotions, what do you need to counter it?" The answer is very simple, "Lots and lots of positive emotions!" And that is part of what I set out to create in myself.

1. Positive Emotions

As mentioned earlier, Dr. Sarno's treatment program includes self-talk, to communicate to the brain (the subconscious mind) a desire to change its behavioral pattern. However, I knew from my studies in psychology that a faster and more effective way of communicating with the mind is through images that produce strong positive emotions.

When I ask the audience which segment of society uses images and strong emotions to affect our minds every day, I always get the following answer: advertisers, of course! Advertisers know that in order to communicate their messages about their products effectively all they have to do is associate them with those images (and sounds) that induce strong positive emotions in consumers, causing them to view those products favorably. This strategy works so well that even harmful products like cigarettes can appear very appealing, especially to young people. Knowing the power of images and strong positive emotions, advertisers spend millions of dollars on a thirty- or sixty-second commercial to impact our minds and our buying decisions every day.

I also knew that Olympic and professional athletes as well as high achievers use visualizations to create strong positive emotions for motivation and high performance. So I planned to take full advantage of this technique and create images of power and strength in my mind with a lot of positive emotions to reverse the effects of negative emotions.

Actually, I had noticed during my long painful ordeal that when I was happy, as when we took a trip to Monterey, I was in less pain. Other back pain sufferers have told me that they have also noticed this correlation.[2]

---

[2] Once I helped a newly married systems analyst who had suffered from three years of pain in his back and pain and numbness in his left leg. As he became aware of the tension-pain connection, he told me that for the few weeks prior his wedding, he was free of pain. He even lifted heavy boxes while moving to a new apartment without any difficulty. It was only after all the joy and excitement of the wedding was

In his book *Anatomy of an Illness,* Norman Cousin described how he realized that negative emotions had caused him a very severe case of arthritis which had left him disabled and in the hospital. Doctors gave him six months to live. But he combined his strong will to live with laughter therapy—he watched funny movies—and was able to reverse the course of the disease and recover. Later he taught and conducted research on mind-body medicine at UCLA's medical school.

So, the first step in my rapid recovery plan was to create a lot of positive emotions.

2. Visualization

Since pain is caused by the mind, the use of imagination is extremely important. We think in pictures. We dream in pictures. A picture is worth a thousand words. Pictures are the language of the mind.

Olympic and professional athletes visualize themselves going through the competition and winning prior to the actual competition. People have achieved amazing results by imagining themselves achieving their goal and then putting their efforts into it. Chapter Six contains some fascinating research on how visualization has helped patients recover faster.

I was going to use imagery and visualization to change the association my mind had made between certain positions or movements and pain. I was going to see myself pain-free in those positions and doing those activities, and getting better and stronger faster and faster.

3. Conditioning

Another aspect to consider was that my body had been conditioned to feel pain under certain conditions, such as sitting, bending, and lifting. This conditioning was like a very bad habit

---

over, and he began dealing with old problems again, that his back and leg pain returned. He recovered by following the rapid recovery plan.

that had to be slowly and steadily broken and replaced by good habits. I was no longer going to let conditioned pain guide my every move and affect the way I went about my daily life. I was going to ignore and fight the pain. I knew that by ignoring a conditioned stimulus—in this case by ignoring pain—I could break the conditioned pattern of feeling pain when sitting, standing, or bending, or in other positions and movements. Ignoring my pain had allowed me to improve immediately and increase my sitting time from about twenty minutes to an hour and a half immediately.

4. Goal Setting

I knew from past experience that when I set a clear goal, got excited about it, and worked toward it, my mind and body gathered and focused all their energies for achieving it. I have often been amazed at how effective setting goals is in helping me to achieve great results. You have probably had similar experiences of setting a goal and obtaining greater results than you had expected.

I had to set short-term goals to increase my mobility and confidence, and long-term goals for achieving complete recovery. So I set short-term goals, such as walking around the apartment without shoes and bending and touching the ground, and long-term goals, such as carrying my children after four weeks and taking karate lessons after eight weeks. I also needed to keep a record of all my accomplishments in order to monitor my progress and determine whether my plan needed any improvements.

5. Hello, Little Subconscious

From my past experience with behavior modification techniques and conditioned response, I knew that the subconscious has the traits of a preschooler. It is the part of us that is impulsive, impatient, and lazy—the part of us that wants to sleep in, eat a lot, watch TV for hours, avoid responsibility, and so on. It is the part of us that gets really excited when we try a new car or a new computer. In other words, it is the child within us.[3]

Imagining that a small misbehaving child within us is causing all this pain turns the subconscious mind, which is something abstract, into something more concrete and easier to understand. This tactic also makes it easier to deal with the subconscious and speed up the process of recovery. Dr. Sarno advises that ignoring the pain will make it go away. Certainly if you ignore a misbehaving child, the child will either stop bothering you or hit you somewhere else to get your attention. But if you ignore a misbehaving child long enough, the child will eventually give up.

Now I will ask you what I ask the audience in my seminars: "What is the fastest way to get a child to do what you want?" That's right! Give him or her candy, ice cream, or some other treat. So as a part of my recovery plan, I was going to use a reward system. Rewards served as a motivating factor for my subconscious to change its negative pattern and move in the positive direction of recovery. Rewards also served as a wonderful way of creating more positive emotions and focusing my mind all day on enjoying a delicious chocolate-covered Häagen–Dazs ice cream bar all day instead of all the things that made me angry, upset, and frustrated.

6. It's Time for Fun

Mental tasks are accomplished much better and more quickly if we are relaxed and enjoy the process. So, in the same way that we can think, learn, and remember better and more rapidly when we are relaxed and enjoy the process, I knew that my recovery would be more rapid if I made it a fun and relaxing experience. It

---

[3] The subconscious mind has many important facets. It is where our habits and emotions are stored. It prepares our body to deal with various situations and act quickly to either run from them or stand and fight. It is the part of us that wakes us up early in the morning when we need to leave for a trip, sometimes even before the alarm goes off. It is a wonderful and complex part of our amazing brain.

is easy to be overwhelmed by worries, frustrations, tension, and pain, and to stop enjoying life!

7. Body over Mind

Furthermore, I planned to be as physically active during the day as possible so that by nighttime I would be extremely tired. A tired body makes it harder for the subconscious to create trouble. Also, by being active and doing things such as stamping my feet while walking, or standing tall and with confidence, the message I sent my mind was one of recovery and health. These strategies are what I call "body over mind."

And, of course, there is prayer. As anyone with chronic pain knows, when you are in pain day after day and feel helpless, faith in God and prayer become very valuable assets. These had certainly helped me get through some very difficult periods, and I believed it was ultimately through God's mercy and help that I would be able to overcome months of pain and disability. After all, I believed it was no coincidence that the answer to many months of searching and prayers came in the mail![4]

These seven components make up the blueprint for my rapid recovery plan. I will explain each component in detail in the chapter on the Nine-Step Rapid Recovery Plan. Since these techniques were ingrained in my mind from my previous experiences of achieving my goals, recovering from my pain was simply a matter of applying these techniques in this situation. I began my recovery with the goal of increasing my mobility, building confi-

---

[4] The health benefits of faith and prayer have received a great deal of publicity and are becoming more accepted in the medical circles. Dr. Larry Dossey's *Healing Words: The Power of Prayer and the Practice of Medicine* (San Francisco: Harper San Francisco, 1993) and Dr. Herbert Benson's *Timeless Healing: The Power and Biology of Belief* (New York: Scribner, 1996) detail extensive scientific studies on the power of prayer and its positive effect on health and healing.

dence in my physical abilities, and returning to normal as quickly as possible.

As mentioned earlier, one of my long-term goals was to be able to carry my six-year-old daughter and four-year-old son in four weeks. It had been more than two years since I had been able to do so. I could not wait for the moment when I could carry them again and play with them as a father would. I was also very excited about the possibility of taking karate lessons in eight weeks. These goals not only made me more excited about the prospect of recovery, but also, once accomplished, would provide me with greater confidence in my physical abilities.

Since TMS pain originates in the brain, the first step, of course, was not just to get mad at my subconscious, but to wage an all-out war on it for all the suffering it had caused me. I imagined myself as a boxer who, after many defeats, had suddenly discovered his opponent's weak point. Now it was my turn to attack the subconscious and win back my health. Previously, every time I thought that a treatment would work, the pain returned with a vengeance and beat me to the ground. But now I was Rocky the boxer, determined to win. I imagined picking up my subconscious and throwing it to the ground over and over again. I threw it so forcefully that the ground shook and made a loud noise; every time I imagined this scene, I felt more powerful, stronger, and victorious. I created so much positive emotion as a result of visualizing this image that it gave me goose bumps.

I also began launching imaginary missiles toward my subconscious and imagined that these missiles—some of them nuclear—were breaking down and destroying the defense barriers the subconscious mind had built to protect itself. These missiles were launched every few minutes for the first day and made me feel powerful and in charge. By the second day I had improved so much that they were no longer necessary.

IMMEDIATE IMPROVEMENTS

I had already begun improving by sitting more than four times longer than usual. Now I set my goal to walk around in the house without shoes; if the preschooler in me cooperated, he would get a scoop of ice cream.[5] My legs were so sensitive that without the cushioning provided by my shoes, the sciatica would flare up immediately. As I began walking through the house with no shoes I felt as if my legs were on fire, but I ignored the burning sensation and kept telling myself with a serious face and a great deal of determination, "I am not going to hurt anymore. I am going to win this one." I continued to walk, one step at a time. After twenty or so painful steps the burning sensation became more tolerable. That night I even dared to take a few careful steps on the kitchen floor where there was no carpet to cushion my step.

I gradually put more pressure on my feet as I walked. I did so to prove to my subconscious that I no longer fell for its defensive tricks and now believed that there was nothing wrong with my legs. I also hit myself on the thighs to accomplish the same goal and to prove that I was not afraid anymore. My children were overjoyed and excited to see me walk without shoes in the house. I also began to bend more and more to pick up things.

When a call came in from the bookstore that my order of *Healing Back Pain* had arrived, I rushed to buy my copy. As I

---

[5] In her book on behavior modification, Karen Pryor wrote about how encouraging and rewarding positive aspects of our behavior (positive reinforcement) can help us become more successful in what we do. She gave the example of a Wall Street lawyer who, instead of cursing himself for making mistakes while playing squash, gave himself a compliment for every good shot and even patted himself on the back when playing alone. Of course, he felt "like a damned fool" doing so at first, but his game improved dramatically and he was able to beat people from whom he could hardly take a point before. Thus, encouraging our inner self can be a very effective means of achieving our goals (*Don't Shoot the Dog,* New York: Simon and Schuster, 1984, pp. 22–23).

was about to step onto the curb from the street with my right leg, I concentrated on making my right knee, which usually felt pain going up even one step, pain-free. This time my right knee did not hurt, but my left knee did! I smiled the smile of victory. This is a characteristic of TMS: The pain moves around once you know the cause. Now that I knew the pain was due to reduction of blood flow, it was easy to ignore it and continue my progress.

I kept my wallet in my back pocket. My buttock area had been so sensitive for so long that I had been unable to keep my wallet in my back pocket. I ignored the irritation caused by the wallet, and it went away.

I did experience severe nausea all day. Knowing that the autonomic nervous system controls the digestive system as well, however, I did not concern myself with it, and the nausea went away. By that night, I was quite proud of the little child in me. I told him how proud I was of him and gave him a scoop of ice cream. We all know how kids love ice cream!

While lying in bed that night, I reviewed my accomplishments for that day. It felt wonderful to have made such rapid improvements and know that finally I was getting better. My goal for the next day was to climb two steps without pain in my knees. I imagined myself doing so over and over, with complete ease and comfort, and becoming stronger and stronger. As you may recall, I had so much pain in my knees and legs that climbing even two steps was quite painful and difficult.

I offered myself a creamy and delicious Häagen-Dazs ice cream bar as a reward and imagined eating it with such great pleasure that my mouth began to water. I knew that such strong, positive emotions can really motivate the subconscious to do the job so that it can get to its reward. I had been following a low-fat diet as a result of my studies of healthy living and rarely had ice cream, so eating a rich, creamy ice cream bar was quite a "childish" thing to do!

The best example of how positive emotions can impact your subconscious is experienced when you are getting ready to go on a vacation. Have you ever noticed that on mornings when you were about to leave for a vacation, you woke up very early, even before the alarm went off? And when you woke up you had so much energy and enthusiasm, none of which was there the day before. What happened? Knowing that something exciting and wonderful is going to happen, your subconscious prepared you to achieve your goal of starting your vacation by waking you up early and with a lot of energy.

Now when you design your recovery plan, if you make it as exciting as going on a wonderful vacation with lots of rewards and pleasurable activities, you can expect your subconscious to help you recover rapidly.

The following is from the log I kept of my recovery.

Monday, March 22

For the first time in about a year I put on a tie. It bothered my neck, but I ignored the irritation, and my neck started feeling better. I said good-bye to my wife and children, who were going to spend the week at my in-laws in Concord for spring break, and went to work.

I walked with a new vigor and sense of life. I felt as if I had died and was coming back to life. Everything looked so beautiful and colorful. I felt like a rusty steam engine that after many months of idleness had just been oiled and serviced and had started to move—a shiny black steam engine with golden trim, strong and powerful. I was picking up speed by the minute and going faster and faster, saying to myself, "I believe I can, I believe I can, I believe I can."

The first thing I did at work, to the surprise of my coworkers, was to throw away the four-inch foam pillow I used to sit on due to tenderness in my buttocks. I changed my ergonomically-designed chair with lumbar support for one that was more like a regular chair. Most of the older chairs in the office had been replaced by chairs with lumbar support to accommodate those with back pain and to support good posture. I thought about how much money is spent unnecessarily on such furniture and equipment. For centuries people lived and worked under much harsher conditions without these ergonomically correct furnishings and without an epidemic of back and neck pain.[6]

I easily reached the lowest file cabinet drawer to remove a file. My ability to do so surprised one of the secretaries, who had helped me just a few days earlier to get a file from the same drawer. I told her and practically everyone at work about Dr. Sarno's book and how it had helped me, hoping that they would also benefit from it.

I did not tell them what the book was about because of the reaction I had received from my friends over the weekend. As I began to improve I started calling friends and relatives and telling them about my discovery. However, the long silent pauses on the other end of the line made me realize most people find the idea that tension causes most back pain difficult to accept. They understood this explanation as meaning that the pain was all in my head. The last thing I wanted my coworkers and my supervisor to think was that I had remained off work for so many months because the problem was in my head!

As I went about my daily routine, I stamped my feet to reinforce in my mind that there was nothing wrong with my legs and that I was no longer afraid of pain. I would also count down from ten as I walked and told my mind to stop the pain when I reached zero. I used certain commands, such as *Drop it,* or *Stop it,* while clenching my fists, squinting my eyes, and making a serious face. These words and expressions create a mental association between these cues and elimination of pain. From my previous studies in psychology, and from personal experience, I knew that this association would make it much easier in the future to stop the pain by a simple command or change in facial expression. The command would bring up all the stored emotions and memories related to the effort I was putting into my recovery, and in a matter of seconds or minutes the pain would be eliminated.

Olympic and professional athletes as well as high achievers use similar techniques prior to a game to put themselves in the

---

[6] My search of relevant literature has yet to reveal any evidence that these types of furniture or wearing support belts prevent back pain.

peak performance zone rapidly. Here, I was applying these techniques to eliminate pain rapidly.

In order to keep my mind focused, at every stoplight I focused my eyes on the light and my mind on God's glory and power. In this way, I showed my gratitude to my Creator for His blessings and created more positive feelings; this also forced my inner child to stay calm and obedient to my conscious mind. We all know that sitting calmly and quietly for a period of time is very difficult for a preschooler. This type of focusing exercise really helps to keep the subconscious in line and is a great way to relax the wondering, anxious mind. This exercise is also considered a form of meditation.[7]

I knew how important it was at this stage of recovery to saturate my mind with as much information as possible on mind/body medicine. So I went to the library and checked out tapes of Norman Cousins' books *Anatomy of an Illness* and *Head First: The Biology of Hope*. In these tapes he discussed his personal experience of overcoming a serious illness through positive emotions as well as the results of many studies conducted at UCLA and other major universities on the effects of positive and negative emotions on health.

Throughout the day I thought how great it would be to climb two or three steps without pain and how wonderful the ice cream bar would taste. I imagined eating it very slowly, relishing and enjoying every bite fully.

That night, I went to the mall to buy a copy of *Healing Back Pain* for my dentist friend. He had had upper back pain for ten years and lower back pain and leg pain for one year. He also suffered from hay fever. After I bought the book, I began to walk through the mall, looking for a stairway in order to climb two to three steps without pain in my knees.

I saw a stairway in a department store. As I approached it, a feeling of complete peace and tranquillity came over me. It was as if I were on a cloud. I began to climb the steps, one after another.

---

[7] These mental exercises and their benefits will be discussed in more detail in Chapter Six.

I had visualized climbing stairs with complete ease so many times for the previous twenty-four hours and had attached to it so much positive feeling that my mind and body had reached optimum performance state for achieving this goal—just as Olympic athletes do prior to a competition.

I began to climb the steps with complete ease and confidence. One, two, three, four, five—I just kept on going up! My eyes were witnessing this amazing feat, but my mind could not believe it. Nothing was hurting—not my knees, nor my piriformis muscles, nor my sciatic nerves. Before I realized it, I was at the top of the stairway. I looked down: *Oh, my God!* I had just climbed seventeen steps! It had been more than a year since I was able to climb so many steps without pain.

For a moment I panicked. I didn't know what to do. It looked like such a long way down. I was not sure whether my knees could take the pressure of going down so many steps yet. There were no handrails to use for support. Finally, after a few moments, I gathered all my courage, took a deep breath, and began my descent—one step at a time. My knees were in pain and shaking, but with each step it became easier. Finally I reached the bottom. What a relief! I had won another battle against pain and come out victorious. I became more confident about my ability to recover, began to stamp my feet again, and continued my march to good health.

I went home and fell on the ground to thank God. But it was still too soon; I had to jump right back up from severe pain in my knees. I did remain true to my promise and gave the little boy in me the promised Häagen-Dazs ice cream bar for the pain-free climb. It was the best-tasting ice cream bar I ever had. I took my time and enjoyed every bite fully. It was a glorious night.

Again, that night before I slept, I reviewed my accomplishments for that day and felt wonderful. I also set my goal for the next day. This time it was for a pain-free upper body. I wanted to feel no pain in my elbows and shoulders. I also wanted to work on the NordicTrack cross-country ski machine we had bought a while back for my wife. I had been dreaming about using it. But I noticed that my excitement about the NordicTrack was childlike. I realized that this machine was really like a toy for the little child inside me. So I told him that if he did not cause me any upper body pain the next day, he could try the NordicTrack as a reward. I also imagined myself doing things such as turning the car's steering wheel, writing with complete ease, and becoming healthier and stronger.

Tuesday, March 23

Since my progress so far had been better than expected, it was time for some positive reinforcement (or encouragement). I decided to stay under the hot shower a few minutes longer this morning and really enjoy it. I also bought a special fruit drink later and told my subconscious this was a little extra reward for being such a good boy yesterday.

While I was at work, one of my coworkers asked about my back, so I bent down and touched the ground to demonstrate how much I had improved. "I'm impressed!" he exclaimed. "It's all because of Dr. Sarno's book," I said, and I advised him to get a copy of *Healing Back Pain.* As I went about doing my job, I had to descend and climb twenty steps at a Kaiser Hospital. Doing so was much easier than the night before.[8]

My elbows and shoulders were 98 percent pain-free. When I went home, I got on the NordicTrack with childlike excitement, and holding on to the handlebar began the foot movement. I felt pain in my knees as I pushed back and forth on the skis, but was able to continue for three minutes. Afterwards, my right sciatic nerve was irritated, but overall it was a good first step. Unfortunately, it was not as much fun as I had hoped, but I had been true to my promise, and that was what really mattered. However, I did

---

[8] While driving I saw a young man limping slowly on the sidewalk. I thought, "Another sciatica sufferer, perhaps?" I was so excited about discovering TMS and my rapid recovery that I wanted to let everyone know and to help whomever I could. So I immediately stopped the car and walked up to him and offered my help. He told me that he was born with a limp! Well, I had tried.

give the little boy in me a scoop of ice cream to make up for the disappointment.

I visited my dentist friend for about an hour or so— something that had been impossible for me to do just three days earlier. He was overjoyed to see me doing so much better. He later told me that just seeing me get well cured his back. I gave him a copy of *Healing Back Pain* as a gift.

I also began listening to tapes on reducing tension through breathing exercises and muscle relaxation. These tapes helped me to reach higher levels of relaxation, and made my subconscious mind more receptive to my conscious commands. I found it quite useful to visualize what I wanted to accomplish while in a state of deep relaxation.

Once again, before I slept, I reviewed my accomplishments for the day and set my goal for an overall pain-free day. I imagined myself working out on the NordicTrack without pain. After months of sleeping with a pillow between my legs and in pain, now I could finally sleep in any position I chose without pain or discomfort. It felt wonderful.

Wednesday, March 24

I worked out three minutes on the NordicTrack without experiencing any pain in my knees or sciatica, loaded and later unloaded the dishwasher, and went up more stairs during work.

During the day, for a moment, I began to doubt whether this recovery was real. Mightn't it all fall apart at any moment and all my pain would come right back? However, since I was breaking through the pain barriers step by step in a carefully designed program, a quick review of my accomplishments replaced my doubts with confidence.[9]

I went for a swim for the first time in more than a year. My knees and legs hurt while I was swimming, but I ignored the pain.

---

[9] For this reason, it is important to keep a record of any progress made. Such a record helps to dispel doubts quickly and build confidence.

However, right after the swim I developed a severe headache. I rarely have headaches, and never after swimming. I realized that this one was another manifestation of tension. Swimming is known both for its physical benefits and as a tension releaser. Being the clever little child that the subconscious is, he tried to give me a headache this time, maybe as an attempt to stop me from swimming. I decided to ignore the headache, for one of the ways to deal with a misbehaving child is to ignore him until he gets tired and quiets down.

However, I thought it would be wise to take a couple of Tylenol PM caplets in order to both quiet the headache and sleep longer that night. The past few days, I had been so tired from all my new activities that I would fall asleep as soon as I went to bed; but I was so excited over my newly restored health that I would wake up in the middle of the night unable to sleep. As I held the caplets in my hand, I imagined that they were just vitamin supplements that I was taking for better health, and I told my subconscious that these had nothing to do with my headache. After all, a preschooler believes what an adult tells him, and the subconscious also believes whatever you imagine.

By now I had become so pain-free going about my daily activities that I did not feel the need to set a goal—and this only four days after I began my recovery. The pain had been so disabling and had lasted so many months that I had often wished I could just wake up one day and it would all be gone. I had dreamed of being able to recover quickly and my dream had come true. I felt fantastic, and grateful for a second chance to live an able life.

Thursday, March 25

By now, I was working out on the NordicTrack twice a day for five minutes and 0.5 km, using only the foot movement. I had difficulty coordinating the hand and foot movements, but my wife was coming back the next day, so I figured I would learn from her how to do it.

Now I could walk long distances without feeling pain. Only a few days earlier, walking more than 100 yards would have meant sciatica and knee pain. I still felt some pain here and there but, as Dr. Sarno noted, we all are entitled to some pain sometime.

I swam 125 yards today, but felt pain in my upper back and had an itch on my thigh. I chose to ignore both of them. I did not scratch myself, but simply ignored the itch, because paying attention to it by scratching it or placing ointment on it would mean that I believed I had an actual skin disorder. This itch was, of course, like the back pain—something that had to be ignored until the subconscious gave up on attracting my attention that way.

Friday, March 26

My wife and children were coming back today. I had not seen them since Monday morning. During the week I had told them over the phone only that I was improving; I did not give them any details. I was planning a big surprise. I washed the dishes, cleaned the kitchen, made a fruit salad, and got the house ready. Just five days earlier, these simple tasks were so painful that I could not do them. I also worked out for six minutes on the NordicTrack.

I usually parked in the street and walked to our building because I could not climb the stairway from the parking area to our apartment. This time I parked in the street; when my family returned I told them I had presents for them, but that I would have to drive the car to the parking lot from the street. So they came down to the parking area and I brought the car over and took the gifts out. Then I walked upstairs with them to our apartment. The kids shouted out of joy. "Look! Daddy can climb the stairs now."

They asked whether I could sit on a chair without a pillow. So I did. They asked whether I could sit on the sofa, so I did that too. They were overjoyed to see me do these things and asked me for a piggyback ride! I told them, "Not yet! But I'm working on it." I asked them whether they would like to go swimming, and of course they loved the idea.

We took the kids to the pool, went out for lunch, walked in the mall, and, to wrap it up, went and visited my dentist friend and his family for two hours. All of that would have been impossible for me just five days earlier.

Tired and happy, I went to sleep that night with a big smile on my face.

Saturday, March 27

I took the kids to a play center for two hours, then to a healthy kids' festival, and had lunch out. That evening, I asked my wife to show me how to coordinate the hand and foot movements on the NordicTrack. But it was still very difficult for me; I almost fell off the machine. Then I imagined myself doing the movements with ease, as if I were taking a brisk walk. A few minutes later, to my wife's amazement, I was able to coordinate the hand and foot movements—another example that shows how effective using one's imagination can be in overcoming physical and mental obstacles.

As I kept going on the NordicTrack, however, I felt a muscle under my stomach get pulled. It was a sudden, painful pull. Now I had to determine whether this pain was from TMS or an actual injury. I walked around for a few minutes. The pain was severe. Then, with determination and firm resolve, I told my subconscious that if this was TMS, it had better stop, and if this was not TMS, my subconscious had better send whatever was necessary to the site to heal it.

Then I went for a nice long walk. The pain gradually subsided, and by the next day I was fine. As far as I was concerned, this incident represented another attempt by my subconscious to stop me from doing what would really help me—exercise to work off my anger and tension.

Sunday, March 28

I did 1 km in seven and a half minutes on the NordicTrack. This morning we went for a walk and visited the health center in our apartment complex. I tried the stationary bike and worked a little on the weight machine. I swam 200 yards: breast stroke, back stroke, and free style. But then I began to experience pain in my wisdom teeth accompanied by a sore throat.

Monday, March 29

I had an appointment with my therapist this morning. This is an important step that may be difficult for some people to take so early in their recovery—returning to locations and meeting with people associated with bad, painful experiences. I had worked extensively for many years to handle such situations, so it was fairly easy to return to the location I had gone to in pain for so many months.

I surprised my therapist by asking him to watch me climb a few steps to see whether I was doing it right. As he watched, I ran up eight or nine steps and walked right back down. He was over-joyed and quite happy that after such a long time I was finally getting well.

I ironed my own shirts that day for the first time in many months. Before, it had been difficult for me to hold and move the iron due to pain in my elbows, and to stand in one place long enough due to sciatica in both legs. Also today, after many months, I was able to cross my legs and sit on the floor.

At night I thought about starting the desensitization process so that words such as disc, sciatic, and tendon, would lose their association with pain. After associating these words with pain and disability for months and years, many people feel pain even thinking about or hearing these words. Desensitization is a fairly simple process during which, under very relaxed conditions, you mention such words or think about them once. Gradually, as thinking about such words becomes easier, you can increase the repetition until saying or hearing these words has no emotional impact. Of course, one can also try rewarding the subconscious. You can promise that you will reward it with ice cream if it lets you desensitize yourself to such words. I myself did not feel the need to do so, since no one I knew at work or at home talked about sciatica, tendinitis, or herniated discs in daily conversation.

I did begin to imagine before sleep that a wall of reinforced concrete was being built around my sciatic nerves and tendons. This wall was absolutely impenetrable by pain agents of the subconscious.

Tuesday, March 30

Besides working on the NordicTrack and swimming, I decided to begin a weight training program. As I prepared to work with the five-pound and ten-pound weights, an upper back muscle suddenly went into spasm. The subconscious definitely has a mind of its own. Somehow it knew that working out with weights would provide me with great confidence and strength, which would make it hard for my subconscious to make me believe that I am weak and use a physical problem as a defense mechanism. So it gave me pain to discourage me from working out.

The weights were light, but for hands that could barely lift a quart of milk ten days earlier, lifting five-pound weights was a great feeling. In fact, just before this, I had tried to pour some water out of a one-gallon container and felt pain in my elbow, pain that persisted. However, I did not let it bother me as I did my triceps exercises. I had a great sense of confidence and freedom.

My sore throat and toothache were gone, but I had a painful pimple on my neck and one on my head. Since I knew that they were caused by tension, I ignored them.

My gastritis was all but gone now. I was able to drink orange juice with no stomach irritation. In fact, for many years, drinking orange juice after a meal used to bother my stomach, but that was no longer a problem either.

Wednesday, March 31

I skied on the NordicTrack for ten minutes and 1.3 km, twice. I cleaned the house, vacuumed the carpets, took a long walk, and worked out with weights. However, I had pain whenever I kneeled to pray. Kneeling is one of my favorite positions when I want to show my gratitude to my Creator; the importance of this activity made me anxious about being able to do it right, so I felt pain. You might notice that it takes a little longer to overcome the pain in movements and positions that are emotionally important to you.

At night, I set my goal not to feel pain when kneeling. So far, I had just used the reward method; but my subconscious was being stubborn, so I had to set a punishment for it. I set fruit yogurt as a reward and cleaning the bathroom as a punishment.

Thursday, April 1

On this day, I noticed an 85 percent improvement in the knees while kneeling. However, this improvement was not good enough.

So I had to clean the bathroom. Interestingly enough, while I was kneeling doing the cleaning, I had no pain, but later, during prayer, I had some pain again. I decided to just ignore it for the time being.

I wrote a letter to Dr. Sarno, thanking him for writing the book and for my restored health.

Friday, April 2

Now I tried to kneel while eating and reading to make this a routine activity. This was sort of a roundabout way of getting myself used to kneeling. I worked out with weights and later took my son to the park. As he was playing, suddenly I felt confident enough to carry him. He was standing on a park bench. I asked him to come close to me, then hugged him and carried him. He was delightfully surprised. This was more than two weeks ahead of schedule.

For over two years I had not been able to lift him. Carrying my children was a goal I had hoped to achieve in one month's time. But by the grace of God, I was able to do it in less than two weeks. Considering that two weeks earlier I could not carry anything heavier than four pounds, that I could now carry my 41-pound son was quite a miracle to me. Obviously I did not become ten times stronger in two weeks, and weak muscles are not the cause of back pain!

That afternoon I decided to surprise my wife and daughter.

While my daughter was jumping on the bed, I grabbed her and carried her to her mother. I told my wife that this girl better learn not to jump on the bed again. Neither of them realized that I was carrying her. I asked if they noticed what was happening, and my daughter shouted with joy. It was a glorious moment.

As I was skiing on the NordicTrack, my nose and lip began to itch, but I told the subconscious to stop it and not to interfere with my exercise. Subsequently, it did stop. The pimples on my neck and head were completely gone today.

Saturday, April 3—Monday, April 5

I skied thirteen minutes on the NordicTrack and finished 2 km. I also worked out with weights. I did the laundry, cleaned and organized closets, and made breakfast.

For the first time in months I attended a community picnic. I met a lot of friends there and spent a long time talking, sitting, and standing. I was able to drive the family van on the freeway. A few minutes of driving the van used to cause me sciatica, but no more.

I noticed that I had no hay fever this year. Usually, by this time of year, being in the park would mean lots of sneezing, a runny nose, and itchy, watery eyes. But this year I was fine.

Some of my friends and coworkers were suffering from hay fever, but I barely sneezed. As soon as I felt an itch in my nose, I realized that it was due to thoughts about matters or people associated in my mind with anxiety or anger; that realization would usually stop the itch. In fact, I even ordered my subconscious to absorb all the mucous generated in my nose, and it did.[10] I avoided blowing my nose or doing anything that would indicate paying attention to that part of my body. This worked well.

My knees had improved quite a bit while kneeling. I found

---

[10] I figured the subconscious mind knows much better than I do how my body's internal system works. So in the same way that it can cause back pain, sciatica, and itchy nose, it also knows how to correct them. I had only to discipline my subconscious and make it obedient to my will; it was the duty of my subconscious to correct the problem.

that imagining a river of blood flowing to my knees or ambulances carrying blood to my knees also helped.

Tuesday, April 6—Friday, April 9

During this period I began climbing stairs two steps at a time, and I played kickball and basketball. I even ran up stairs with no problem at all, and jogged for ten minutes. I took the kids to the park to ride their bikes for the first time in months. I felt quite well, with very little or no pain in my daily activities. I also met with the YMCA fitness instructor, who gave me some valuable information on proper exercise techniques with weights and recommended Covert Bailey's book Fit or Fat as good reading.[11]

I called a professor friend of mine to give him the good news of my recovery. He had been suffering from asthma for years and recently was operated on for hiatus hernia; both of these conditions are TMS equivalents. He told me that recently he had become allergic to broccoli, and eating it had brought on an asthma attack. I explained to him the relationship between tension and physical symptoms and told him that his "allergy" to broccoli was caused by association.[12] My friend's asthma attack was due to

---

[11] Covert Bailey's series of books and tapes on proper nutrition and exercise are excellent sources of information for staying fit. His lectures are filled with facts and humor. Two of his latest books are *The New Fit or Fat* (Boston: Houghton Mifflin, 1991) and *Smart Exercise* (Boston: Houghton Mifflin, 1994).

[12] Association, as a part of conditioning, plays an important role in physical symptoms. Aside from the conditioned response of pain to certain positions and movements, specific factors within our environment can become associated with pain or illness. These factors have to be of significant concern, consciously or subconsciously. A very well-known one is cold weather, but the associated factor can be anything else the mind considers significant. Association is very important to understand because it explains why some people have seasonal back pain. Association can happen with any of the TMS equivalents as well and explains why some people develop allergic reactions, rash, or asthma to foods, locations, or other factors that had never previously caused them problems.

negative emotions. Since the attack came when he was eating broccoli, the sight, smell, and taste of broccoli became associated with the attack, and now broccoli had begun to act as a cue for my friend's subconscious mind to initiate an asthma attack, a conditioned response.

Saturday, April 10—Tuesday, April 20

I had a dentist appointment. My dentist had read *Healing Back Pain* and was working on his hay fever. We discussed how some mouth- and tooth-related problems with unknown causes, such as sensitive teeth, could be other TMS equivalents.

I wrestled with my kids, carried them on my back, and organized the lower kitchen cabinets, which involved lots of squatting and reaching in low areas. I had some lower back discomfort, which I worked out by wrestling with the kids again.

During this period, I increased my workouts on the Nordic-Track to twenty-six minutes and 4.3 km. I swam 600 yards and noticed that my sinuses, which are usually congested, had cleared up completely—probably because the increase in the length of my exercise time allowed more tension to be released and my body to become more relaxed. As the mind and body reach higher levels of relaxation, the more established patterns of tension-related symptoms are broken, leading to their disappearance.

Wednesday, April 21

One month ago, I could barely walk 100 yards or go up two steps. Today, I began taking karate lessons. Ever since I saw my first Bruce Lee movie I had always wanted to become a black belt. I took two semesters of karate in college but was always too busy to continue studying karate after that. During my disability I had felt guilty that I had not taken advantage of my health and continued studying karate while I still could. I thought that with two degenerated discs and osteoarthritis of the spine, I would never be able to study karate again. But now I could—and four weeks ahead of schedule.

The self-discipline and self-defense techniques in karate are of great benefit, both physically and mentally. Furthermore, all that kicking, punching, and screaming is a good way of working off tension. I did the kicks, punches, and other movements, all of which caused some pain, but none of which stopped me. I knew that when I got used to the movement I would not feel pain later. I also swam 600 yards.

Thursday, April 22—Sunday, April 25

I started working out on a universal weight machine, working on all the major muscle groups. I also worked on the Nordic-Track for twenty-four minutes and 3.6 km.

My mother came for a visit. She was overjoyed to see my improvement. When she saw me carry the children her eyes filled with tears of joy. However, she advised me not to tell anyone about this mind over body stuff, lest people think I was crazy!

We decided to take a trip to Monterey for a weekend getaway. I did the hour-and-a-half drive to Monterey for the first time in more than a year. During the trip I felt great, despite the usual tension between my mother and me. However, as soon as we returned, my back became stiff and the pain began, but now I knew it was due to all the tension I had been under for the past few days. Interestingly enough, I felt no pain while driving to Monterey and looking forward to an enjoyable weekend!

I was not surprised at this episode of back pain. It had been a little more than a month since my recovery had begun, and I knew that certain circumstances that are subconsciously associated with a great deal of tension will cause pain. Overcoming the pain was only a matter of facing those situations, dealing with the pain, and moving on.

It is common to experience an episode of back pain when returning from a vacation. For most people, coming back from vacation means returning to problems and responsibilities. So, as they get closer to home, the pain begins; people usually attribute it to a long drive, a bad seat, or carrying heavy suitcases. As discussed earlier, the reverse of this situation can also happen; sometimes repressed anger, anxiety, and worries get a chance to manifest themselves only when a person is on vacation.

Monday, April 26

This morning I had more pain in my back than I had the day before. It was so bad that if I made one wrong move I would scream from the pain, but I did not let it stop me. I swam 400 yards and did twenty-eight minutes for 4 km on the NordicTrack. Despite the pain, I lifted my kids and tried to act as though nothing were wrong.

Tuesday, April 27—Friday, April 30

My back was 90 percent better and was free of pain just two days after the pain had begun. I continued my karate lessons and weightlifting program. I did not have time for swimming anymore, so I stopped it for now.

Saturday, May 1—Thursday, May 6

I played tennis with a friend who had been suffering from pain in his back and right hand for many months. He was a software engineer who had been to many doctors and had received many treatments. I had already explained TMS to him and put him on my program. As we played tennis he felt pain in his right hand, but he was determined to get back into playing tennis again. So he hit harder and harder. The pain in his right hand got worse and began to radiate up his arm. After a few more shots, his left hand began to hurt. He had never had pain in his left hand before! He too realized it was TMS all along, and recovered.

As I was looking for more information on reducing tension, I came across a book titled *Tension Turnaround*.[13] The book men-

---

[13] Faelton, Sharon and David Diamond, *Tension Turnaround* (Emmaus, Pa.: Rodale Press, 1990). This book provides strategies for dealing with tension, anger, and stress in everyday life and under dif-

tioned back pain as a common manifestation of tension, and family problems as the major cause of it. The book explained how tension produces many physical changes in our bodies. For example, due to tension most of us do not breathe deeply, as babies do. Instead of deep abdominal breathing, most people breathe only at chest level, so that they do not make full use of their lung capacity. Deep, abdominal breathing helps to relax the entire body and counteracts many physical manifestations of tension.

Although I did some breathing exercises daily while listening to relaxation tapes, when I began to do the deep breathing techniques I noticed resistance on the part of my subconscious; my heart would beat faster and I would feel anxious. Obviously, deep breathing meant breaking a well-established habit that the subconscious did not want broken. It took a few sessions of practicing the technique over a period of a few days for it to become relaxing.

Friday, May 7

I was examined by an ophthalmologist for my first eye exam since I had moved. For fourteen years I had been diagnosed as slightly farsighted with astigmatism in the left eye and needing glasses for reading. Now the ophthalmologist diagnosed me as slightly nearsighted and not needing any glasses. Because I felt that he had hurried through the examination and because his diagnosis contradicted those of five other optometrists and an ophthalmologist, I called the clinic for another examination. This time another ophthalmologist examined me and gave the same diagnosis. "You are young and there is no reason why you should need glasses," the doctor said. I was glad, but puzzled!

Could it be that at some point in my life, as a result of tension, my eyes had not been at their best on the day they were examined, so that the optometrist prescribed glasses for me, which I then became conditioned to require? I usually could read for a few

---

ferent circumstances. It also has a chapter on back pain and its relationship to tension and stress.

minutes before my eyes felt strained, and once, when my glasses were lost for three weeks, I developed headaches and eyestrain when I had to read. But now, armed with my newly gained knowledge about tension's effects and assurances from two doctors, I began to read without glasses and experienced no problems. In fact, I have not needed eyeglasses since.[14]

Later I remembered the circumstances under which I had to get my first glasses. When I finished my course in psychology, I had tried to resolve my parents' conflicts and bring some peace and harmony to our lives. However, my efforts were not appreciated and caused even more problems. During this very tense period I began to experience eyestrain and headaches while studying, which resulted in a visit to the optometrist and my reading glasses.

As I took my children to the park this Friday afternoon, I realized suddenly that I had been so busy today that I had completely forgotten how disabled I was just a few weeks earlier—how I had to hold a cup of water with both hands in order to get a drink, and how even that action had caused pain. I began to weep, partly from sorrow and partly from joy. As planned and calcu-

---

[14] Later I discovered Dr. William Bates's book *Better Eyesight Without Glasses* (New York: Henry Holt, 1971), in which he explains the incorrect diagnosis and approach by the medical establishment to eye refractions. Using simultaneous retinoscopy, he was able to demonstrate in thousands of patients that tension can cause an error in refraction (e.g., nearsightedness). In fact, he points out that the lens has very little to do with the refraction error. It is the eye muscles that shorten or lengthen the eye for better vision. I found Dr. Bates' arguments to be almost exactly the same as Dr. Sarno's, except that Dr. Bates' apply to the eye instead of the back. He says to ignore all the dos and don'ts, such as the advice not to read in dim light, and with a relaxed mind, an active imagination, and a number of eye exercises, one can get rid of the need for glasses. Of course, I would add that ordering one's mind to relax the eyes for better vision helps too. I highly recommend Dr. Bates' book; I also recommend *The Art of Seeing* by Aldous Huxley, a man who suffered from near-blindness and, using Dr. Bates' methods, recovered completely.

lated as my recovery had been, the reality of it still overwhelmed me at times.

Saturday, May 8—Monday, May 10

I had to have some costly car repairs done, which were a source of stress, and I noticed that my hay fever was back. The local news was filled with stories about the high pollen counts that had resulted from a rainy winter following seven years of drought, and the expcted allergic reactions to all the pollen. Almost everyone I met was sneezing and suffering from allergies.

I knew I had to fight back again. I kept telling my subconscious to stop the allergy attacks, but I was not having much success in controlling the hay fever. It was time to bring out the treat for the little boy in me. I promised him before sleep that if I did not sneeze at all the next day, I would give him a Häagen-Dazs ice cream bar as a reward.

Tuesday, May 11

On nine separate occasions my nose began to itch, but as soon as I thought about a luscious, creamy Häagen-Dazs ice cream bar, the itching stopped, and I did not sneeze at all the entire day. That evening I bought the little boy in me his reward and thanked him for his cooperation. Of course, the reason this effort was so effective was due to my previous positive experience with this approach and the trust that I had built between my conscious and subconscious mind by being true to my promises.

Wednesday, May 12

I sneezed twice today, but another promise of ice cream stopped any other attacks. Except for an occasional sneeze or two, I was fine the rest of the allergy season.

Friday, May 21

I moved the NordicTrack resistance to level 4 and did twenty-eight minutes and 3.1 km. I wrote a letter to Dr. Sarno about my two months of progress.

Shortly after I finished the letter, I went to the weight room and worked on the universal weight machine. While doing the lat pull-down exercise,[15] I felt pain in my right shoulder (the deltoid muscle). I ignored the pain and continued with the rest of my routine. I was fine till the next day when, ten minutes into skiing on the NordicTrack, my shoulder began to hurt again. I ignored the pain and continued for another twenty minutes with my other exercises, which included twenty push-ups. During these exercises, my shoulder did not hurt, but afterward I began to feel a tingling sensation going down my right arm. The rest of the day I felt pain when steering the car or doing anything that used that muscle, but I noticed that when I talked and laughed with friends, swam, or concentrated on doing something else, I was not aware of the pain or the tingling sensation.

I felt that my plan to discuss some serious, troublesome issues with my wife had something to do with the pain. So there was possibly some manifestation of TMS involved here. In fact, I experienced some left groin and sciatic pain also as I did my squats on the weight machine, but that pain was an old trick and I was able to stop it quickly.

I continued to wonder whether some actual physical injury had occurred because I moved up to heavier weights too early. Was it possible that the injury was a minor one and that my mind was blocking out the pain? And if I went back to weightlifting too soon, might I risk a serious injury? Finally I decided it was most likely a case of TMS for the following reasons:

1. Emotional factors seemed to be involved.
2. I had no pain or discomfort after the workout till the next day and ten minutes into my exercise.
3. If an actual physical injury was involved, it would have caused pain at the time and immediately afterward.
4. An actual physical injury would have continued to hurt when I was enjoying the company of friends or taking a swim.

[15] This exercise involves sitting and pulling down with both hands on a steel bar attached to weights.

5. The right shoulder showed no signs of redness or swelling.

For these reasons, the pain appeared to be a case of TMS.

Just listing the reasons that I believed this was TMS brought about an 80 percent reduction in my pain, and shortly after, when I read of a related case that Dr. Sarno had mentioned in his book (p. 75), I recovered completely and went immediately to the weight room.

The real reason for the pain was a deep-seated anxiety that I might hurt myself during the weightlifting. This anxiety was reinforced by various books on the topic that discuss the possibility of serious injury during weightlifting. Certainly, after such a long period of disability, the last thing I wanted to do was to cause myself some real injury.

After this incident, I also realized that I had been a little too careful in my daily tasks, saving my energy for when I exercised. Because I was babying myself to some extent, I felt some pain in my elbows and knees. I decided that before this whole ordeal I was, overall, a pain-free person, and that was how I wanted to live again.

I set my mind on being absolutely pain-free. By stamping my feet while walking and putting more physical effort into whatever I did, I became completely pain-free.

Saturday, May 22—Tuesday, June 1

It had been about a month since I had gone swimming. At that time 600 yards in thirty minutes was my limit. So I decided to go for a swim and see how far I could swim in thirty minutes. To my surprise, I was able to swim 900 yards quite easily. Being able to do so was a positive consequence of cross-training. I also passed my first test in karate and qualified for an orange belt.

Wednesday, June 2

I woke up with a sore throat. I had had another sore throat recently that had disappeared in two days. So I decided to ignore the pain and continue my exercise program. After weightlifting and karate, I felt exhausted at night.

Thursday, June 3—Sunday, June 6

On Thursday morning I woke up feeling very tired. I had a sore throat and was generally feeling sick. I reduced my exercise program to half, but by Saturday, June 5, I was really ill. This time it was the real thing: sore throat, coughing, earache, sinus congestion, and fever.

Monday, June 7—Thursday, June 24

The doctor prescribed antibiotics and ordered bed rest.[16] I noticed that my back was beginning to hurt. My wife and dentist friend also came down with colds and their backs began to hurt!

It is very common for back-pain sufferers to experience a return and increase in severity of pain when experiencing other ailments. I could see that having to lie down most of the time could trigger a conditioned response and bring back old memories of back pain. It could also be that focusing one's attention on the body brings back the back pain. Of course, a cold or flu can come on fairly quickly and disrupt one's routine or plans. This disruption can create tension and can bring about back pain.

In a way, I was happy to get sick and have the back pain now, because any time a conditioned response is broken, the chances of the response developing again become less or even nil. So the sooner I broke this conditioned response, the fewer problems I would have later. Also, I had more than two glorious months of healthy, active life to be grateful for. I thanked God that I did not get sick during that crucial period when I had just learned about TMS.

I wondered whether my subconscious would attempt to take

---

[16] According to *The Doctors' Book of Home Remedies* (Emmaus, Pa.: Rodale Press, 1990), a positive attitude about the body's ability to heal itself and an active imagination can mobilize the immune system forces to fight a cold (p.145). I have tried this technique and found it quite helpful.

advantage of the situation. I noticed that at times I could stop the tingling sensation in my throat and prevent a cough by ordering the sensation to stop. Although initially both my ears hurt, after nearly two weeks of taking antibiotics my right ear was well but my left ear continued to hurt.

Because my attention had been focused on my earache, I wondered whether this pain was actually a case of temporomandibular joint syndrome (TMJ), where the jaw joint, which is next to the ear, feels tender and painful. According to Dr. Sarno, this jaw pain is another manifestation of TMS. I knew that until my wife and I had worked out our differences, we would probably both experience some manifestation of TMS or its equivalents. In fact, my wife was suffering from shoulder pain during this period.

I went to see my family doctor to make sure this was not a case of some antibiotic-resistant bacteria causing the pain. He said my ear looked fine. I asked him to check for TMJ. When he pressed on my right jaw joint I felt severe pain, although otherwise it was not painful. I remembered Dr. Sarno mentioning that in cases of TMS the pain can be felt in other areas when related muscles are pressed, although one does not usually feel pain in that particular location. Relieved that I did not have a persistent infection, I was free of TMJ pain shortly thereafter.

Friday, June 25—Saturday, July 31

It took some time to regain my strength and get back into my exercise routine and karate, but I eventually did. During a conversation about tension with a friend, he mentioned that when he is under a lot of stress he gets constipated and later develops severe headaches. I wondered whether it is also possible to reverse constipation due to stress. I follow a low-fat, high-fiber diet and normally do not experience constipation. But when I did a few days later, I realized it was due to tension and ordered my subconscious to make things happen. And sure enough, in less than a minute I was fine.

I also discovered that hiccups are a TMS equivalent. I had just finished dinner when I received a stressful phone call. Shortly afterward I began to hiccup, but knowing about tension and physical symptoms, I quickly made the connection and ordered my mind to stop. The hiccups stopped immediately.

On July 31, I passed the test for the next belt in karate and received a gold (yellow) belt.

August—Present

Nowadays, I rarely experience TMS because I have learned how to manage stress better, but when I do feel TMS-related pain, I am able to eliminate it very quickly. Since I have a calm personality, on the conscious level I still cannot measure how angry or upset certain incidents make me. The physical symptoms that I experience later help me measure the emotional impact of a stressful situation. I am still the same easygoing person I have always been, but I no longer hesitate to let people know that I cannot be pushed beyond my limits. With prayer and meditation, regular exercise, a healthy diet, regular activities that I enjoy, and, above all, better communication with my wife, I have been able to manage stress and tension much better and lead a much happier and more enjoyable life.

5

THAT'S LIFE

*A*t this point, you might be wondering what were the sources of anger and tension in my life that had caused me to become almost totally disabled. As a rule, I do not like to discuss my personal problems. I believe most people have enough problems of their own; they can do without hearing about mine. However, I must make an exception in this case and explain some aspects of my life and the circumstances that caused my back pain—circumstances that are unfortunately very common in today's society. I hope this short account will help elucidate the relationship between repressed negative emotions and physical symptoms more clearly.

GROWING UP WITH TENSION

After I finished reading *Healing Back Pain,* I began to analyze the sources of anger and tension in my life. As I was growing up, my parents were constantly arguing and fighting, and I realized now why I had suffered from acne, hay fever, and heart palpitation for many years.

In a family where an argument or an outright fight between the parents occurs almost every day, children feel helpless, anxious, angry, and frustrated as they watch two people they love who are never at peace. Facing such an unpleasant, hopeless situation, children's only defense is to repress their negative emotions and carry on as if nothing terrible is happening, while constantly dreaming of a life filled with love and peace at home instead. My brothers and I treated the fights as routine and ignored them, but in fact we were hurting.

STRATEGIES FOR A BETTER LIFE

My first break from my tension-filled family life came when I went to college. In my freshman psychology class I learned how to use behavior modification techniques, goal setting, and positive thinking to change my life for the better. I learned how habits are formed and that indeed we are creatures of habit. My psychology teacher helped us understand how to apply visualization, conditioning, positive and negative reinforcement, and other behavior modification techniques to form good habits and overcome bad ones.

Imagery and Visualization

My instructor taught us that the inception of every action is in the mind. It is the mind that conceives the action first, whether consciously or unconsciously; only afterward is the action carried out by the body. The most routine physical movement, such as walking, was at one time in our lives—when we were babies or while recovering from an injury or illness—quite a challenge, requiring conscious effort and coordination to accomplish.

As a result of conditioning and repetition, walking is a routine part of most people's lives and is done with no conscious effort. We do not need to think about how we are going to take each step; we simply decide to walk to a certain place and we do. The same is true for driving a car or riding a bicycle. At first we need to make conscious efforts to learn the skills involved, but later we do these activities with no need to think about every movement.

So it is vital to consider the mind/body interaction in

initiating or developing a desired action or behavior. The most effective way to communicate with our minds is through images and feelings; so imagery and visualization play a crucial role. By using these techniques to form the proper images in our minds and feel the appropriate feelings prior to and during formation of a desired habit or while overcoming an obstacle in our lives, we prepare ourselves mentally and emotionally, and the required physical changes become easier. For example, if you want to begin a regular jogging program or to become a good public speaker, you must find a quiet place where there are no distractions, take a few deep breaths, close your eyes, and for a few minutes imagine yourself doing those things step by step and in complete detail from start to finish.

You must be able to picture every detail, from the clothes you wear to how sunny and nice that day would be—feel the warm sun on your face as you jog and smell the wildflowers on the jogging trail, or see and hear the cheering crowd as you begin your speech. The more vivid and colorful your images, the more clear the sounds, and the more real those feelings are, the easier it will be for you to make the change. You must see yourself performing these new activities with complete ease, success, and satisfaction. Set your goals high and see yourself winning a major jogging competition or giving a wonderful speech in a large auditorium, enthralling thousands.

Imagine yourself seeing the sights and hearing the sounds. Experience the feelings—all the emotions you associate with winning and success. Images and emotions are what determine how we feel about things. It is our feelings, primarily feelings of pain and pleasure, that drive us toward certain behaviors and keep us from others.

Imagery and visualization are very powerful techniques and can bring about amazing results. They are also used to overcome many phobias and other mental obstacles that can hinder our growth and capabilities.

Time for Action

The second stage to forming a new habit is to take action by making gradual changes in small, planned steps toward attaining the desired results, and continuing until you succeed. You must write out a complete detailed plan with specific goals and deadlines for achieving them. For example, you learn about the benefits of regular exercise and decide to begin jogging five days a week. The first day you may simply put on your jogging shoes and walk around the house for a few minutes; the next day walk a few minutes toward the nearest track; on the third day go to the track and look around; on day four, walk around the track once; over the next few days begin to jog, and then increase the distance.

This approach may take longer and initially may not seem as rewarding as going for a two-mile jog the first day would, but it will allow your mind and body to adjust to your desired new habit much more easily. It is much more likely that you will remain committed to your exercise program if you use this approach, rather than becoming just an occasional jogger or a weekend athlete.

Positive Association

This new habit can become even more a part of your routine—and an enjoyable part at that—if it is associated with rewards and positive reinforcement as each stage of the plan is completed. In fact, positive and negative associations with certain behaviors, incidents, and products play an important role in determining our attitude toward them.[1]

Your inner child—that lazy part of you that does not want to jog—will look forward to jogging when completion of your

---

[1] Advertisers know the powerful impact positive associations have on our minds. That is why tobacco advertisements and beer commercials use magnificent scenery, beautiful settings, and attractive models or popular athletes to associate such products with symbols of health, wealth, and happiness.

exercise could mean a scoop of ice cream or a nonfat frozen yogurt. You can also give yourself positive reinforcements such as positive self-talk and even a pat on the back to provide the needed encouragement. Of course, jogging or whatever new habit you form gradually becomes a part of your routine, and eventually you do not need to reward the subconscious for it.

So even though you might have been too lazy or too busy to start a regular exercise program initially, in just a few weeks you can adapt to this new addition to your daily routine. As you begin to reap the benefits of regular exercise and feel stronger and healthier, you will actually begin to like it. You will even feel guilty if you miss an exercise session without a valid reason.

In my case, before I went to college I had never been athletic and had always found it too difficult to exercise regularly. So I decided to use what I had learned in my psychology class. Using visualization and following a simple action plan, in a few short weeks I was jogging regularly, and not long afterward I added swimming and lifting weights to my exercise routine. I recognized the great value of behavior modification techniques, and I liked the results so well that I decided to apply these techniques to other things I found difficult to do, such as studying chemistry. I decided to make studying for my freshman chemistry course an easy and pleasurable experience!

ENJOYING CHEMISTRY!

I first visualized myself studying my chemistry book page by page, enjoying myself, and eventually getting an A on my final exam. I could feel how proud my parents and my instructor were to see my good grade. I also visualized to myself how horrible I would feel if I did not pass with a good grade, how upset both I and my parents would be, and how such an outcome could ruin my plans for the future.

Now it was time to take action. I held the book for a few minutes. Later I looked at some of the pages, and I took a sip of orange juice as my reward for every page studied. By doing so I developed a positive association with, and good feelings for, chemistry. I studied page after page, until I found myself learning more and more about chemistry; and as I developed a better comprehension of the subject, I actually began to like it. Of course, the A-minus I received in chemistry that semester certainly helped reinforce my good feelings for it. I have to mention that I also set up certain punishments, such as cleaning the bathroom, as backup, just in case my lazy inner child decided to keep me from studying; but most of the time we were on good terms and rewarding it was all I had to do to get its cooperation.

BREAKING BAD HABITS

The same principles apply to breaking bad habits. If you smoke, first visualize yourself smoking less and less every day with the end result being a smoke-free life and a healthier, stronger you. You should also visualize the worst consequences of this destructive habit: see yourself in a hospital bed with emphysema, hooked up to an oxygen machine, lonely and sad, in pain, and gasping for air.

In both cases make yourself feel the intense pain and pleasure each result can bring you. Relish the thought of reaching your goal and rewarding yourself. Feel how hard the punishment will be for failure. Hear the sounds and smell the smells associated with each outcome, and realize the full impact of quitting or continuing this habit. Now plan for a gradual reduction in the number of cigarettes you smoke. Set rewards for each stage of recovery and punishments for lack of progress. Give yourself positive self-talk and encouragement. Using the other techniques I've discussed, with realistic expectations for your progress, you could break this habit in a few weeks.

This method is far more effective than quitting cold turkey for a few days or weeks out of guilt, anger, shame, or frustration, and then returning to the same old habit. Of course, because we are creatures of habit, bad habits must be replaced with good ones that provide substitutes for most of the benefits lost as a result of the change. If you smoke to cope with stress, then you should consider other means of relaxation, such as regular breathing exercises or a daily walking program, instead. Also, make things easy for yourself at the beginning by holding a pen between your fingers and chewing gum to keep your hand and mouth busy while you are quitting, and reward yourself for doing the right thing.

BE REALISTIC

It is very important to have realistic expectations about your progress. If you set your expectations too high, it is easy to be disappointed and give up on what comes to seem an impossible task. In contrast, reasonable goals that are easy to attain help you build confidence in your ability to conquer your bad habits and your lazy subconscious and reach your goal. Even if progressing in small steps means it takes you two weeks or a month longer to succeed, so what? You are not competing with anyone, and gradual improvement is much better than giving up. And if while you are making a change you relapse—by smoking a cigarette or missing an exercise session—remember that you are only human, and human beings have many shortcomings. Don't give up. Analyze the events and factors that led to your slip, learn from them, and try not to make the same mistake again.

A NEW OUTLOOK ON LIFE

These techniques and concepts opened a whole new way of looking at life for me. At the time I was an introverted seventeen-year-old, with low self-esteem, a poor self-image, and very little self-confidence—a weakling suffering from allergies and colds most of the year. But now I understood that what I was, for the most part, was the product of my environment and many years of conditioning, and I could manipulate the processes that conditioned me to become who I was, in order to become who I wanted to be.

So I decided to act as my own psychotherapist and began to take charge of my life. I used visualization, conditioning, goal-setting, association, positive and negative reinforcement, desensitization, positive self-talk, focusing, and other means to concentrate all my thoughts and energy to reach my goals and build my self-esteem, self-confidence, and willpower. I became a determined, persistent, highly motivated, and goal-oriented person. I was able in a very short time to achieve my goals and accomplish things I had only dreamt about, from public speaking to fifty pushups a day.

I had practiced visualization and the other techniques so much that I could go through the steps of modifying a certain behavior very quickly and make the improvements I wanted— sometimes simply by telling my subconscious what to do. This previous experience with my subconscious was very helpful in my understanding of Dr. Sarno's approach and in challenging TMS. Of course, despite all these improvements I was far from being perfect; I had, and still do have, many shortcomings—as my friends and relatives can tell you.

LIFE-ENHANCING PRINCIPLES

Now that I had learned about how much my environment had affected my personality and behavior, and how easy it was to change many aspects of both, I began to question and examine all my ideas, beliefs, and behaviors. I did not want to be limited by my upbringing and wanted to reshape my life for the better.

I knew that whatever beliefs, principles, and behaviors I chose were based on my knowledge at the time, and I must always be willing to reexamine and improve or abandon these beliefs and behaviors as new information became available. Thus I tried to learn more and increase my knowledge about matters that were of great concern to me by reading about them and interviewing those with more experience and knowledge. In this way I hoped to learn from the experiences of others and not repeat their mistakes or try to reinvent the wheel.

As I learned more I noticed that, unfortunately, lack of openness to new ideas and solutions appeared to be one major reason for the failure of individuals, companies, and nations to succeed. History is filled with many cases in which the truth had reached people, but their lack of openness to a new way of thinking—or their inability to look at a situation or problem in a new light—caused them to miss out on great opportunities, to endure unnecessary pain and suffering, or even to bring about their own destruction.

A good historical example is the ridicule and resistance Louis Pasteur faced when he showed that doctors' washing their hands and instruments before delivering babies would dramatically reduce the rate of childbirth fever and mortality. Unfortunately, shortsightedness and resistance to new ideas continue in the modern age, as the medical community has yet to recognize the significance of Dr. Sarno's diagnosis, and by resisting and ignoring it allows millions to suffer in agony.

Thus, I promised myself always to keep an open mind in every matter and examine all the evidence prior to making a judgment, leaving open the possibility of revising my decision as new information becomes available. This principle of open-mindedness and flexibility in thinking has helped me on many occasions. It was a combination of this and other such empowering principles, and my fruitful experiences with behavior modification techniques, that helped me to persist in my search for a cure, prompted me not to disregard TMS, and made it possible for me to overcome months of back pain and disability so quickly.

A CLEAR MIND

Some people find it mentally and emotionally safer to remain ignorant or to view difficult situations through rose-colored glasses and avoid facing the truth. Knowing that mental defenses such as denial and regression—which are natural reactions to unpleasant circumstances—can keep a person from facing the truth of a situation, I did my best to detect such defenses in myself and stop them or shorten the length of time I experienced them. After all, our actions begin in our minds, and a clear mind that acts based on reality and true knowledge is a great asset. Anyone can achieve many wonderful things in life by being open-minded and willing to learn and act upon true knowledge. It is just a matter of having the correct knowledge and the courage and discipline to act upon it.

TYPE A PERSONALITY

I also learned in my psychology class that our personalities, thoughts, and emotions affect our health. I learned that the Type A personality, characterized by impatience, hostility, and competitiveness, was found to contribute to heart attacks. I was taught that negative feelings such as anger and anxiety can cause ulcers and high blood pressure. So I decided that as long as I was modifying my behaviors for the better, I should modify my personality and character as well for a healthier and more peaceful life. I tried to become more patient and easygoing, and less inclined to become angry or frustrated easily. Actually, I did such a good job conditioning myself to repress my anger, frustrations, anxieties, and other negative emotions that I did not realize how angry and frustrated I was prior to and during my back problems.

Of all the courses I took in college, this one course in psychology had the greatest impact on my life. The concepts and techniques I learned have helped me immensely and continue to be of great benefit to me.

MARRIED LIFE

After I had finished college and had worked for a while, I was introduced to a young lady who I thought at the time would make the perfect wife. During our courtship we discussed various aspects of marriage and parenthood. We seemed to agree on everything. However, after we got married, we realized there were still many matters about which we differed. Over the years we argued about them and, like most couples, later made up. As we were blessed with two healthy, beautiful children, a girl and a boy, we avoided arguments for the children's sake and kept our anger and frustrations in. However, being unaware of what repressed anger can do, we began to suffer a number of ailments.

I experienced pain in my jaw joints (TMJ) and upper back. My wife suffered from headaches, high blood pressure, and lower back pain.

These manifestations of tension got worse, at least for me, when a close relative advised me that for a more peaceful and harmonious family atmosphere, it would be better not to argue and to keep issues that angered me to myself.

MY BACK PAIN

The conflicts at home, combined with commuting 100 miles a day, being too tired to be a good father, and demands from my parents, all contributed to cause my back pain.

Unfortunately, these problems became worse, as I felt no one took my back pain seriously and everyone continued to expect me to meet their demands and expectations as before. I have myself to blame as well, as I did not complain much about my back pain, which made others think it was not that severe. So I ended up accommodating others beyond my capacity, both physically and emotionally; the result was more pain.

My bad experience with the first doctor caused me more tension and led to sciatica in my right leg. Now I know why it was four days after I felt pain doing the stretches before that sciatica began. My sense of job responsibility made me tolerate the pain and commute 100 miles a day to work. But as soon as I felt I could relax, all the repressed anger I felt toward the doctor manifested itself during my sleep and I woke up with sciatica in my right leg.

As I have mentioned, physical pain related to TMS is often a very apt manifestation of the emotional pain we feel. I hated commuting, so my subconscious found a way to get me out of it: numbness in my right leg—the leg that presses on the gas pedal! I ended up staying with a friend and not commuting anymore.

I have seen this same phenomenon in so many people: the professor who coughs and has to take breaks from her lectures, so she can rest; the programmer whose hand hurts and cannot work.

Getting back to my story, I was hesitant to file for workers' compensation due to career concerns and my reluctance to be thought of as having a chronic debilitating condition. When I finally did so and my duties were modified to accommodate my condition, my tension and anxiety were actually multiplied. I felt inadequate at my job for not being able to perform all my responsibilities. I was trying to get well as fast as possible, and the modification of my duties became another source of anxiety.

More Pain

My experiences with the first physical therapy group and later with the orthopedic surgeon caused more tension. My piriformis muscle that received the cortisone shot became the focus of all my anger toward the doctor who had misled me into believing that the shot would be a painless, wonderful experience. The muscle also became conditioned to feel pain. It took seven months before I could actually stretch the muscle without experiencing a spasm and consequent sciatica. But it remained tender until I learned about TMS.

My knees began to hurt shortly after my wife returned to her job as a systems analyst and we had to place our son in day care. He was four years old at the time and quite attached to his mother. He cried a lot and resisted being left at the day-care center. I was also quite concerned about what all this would do to him mentally and emotionally, and frustrated over my own inability to do anything about it. That was when I began to have pain in my knees. Of course, it was diagnosed by the doctors and my therapist as tendinitis.

Embarrassingly enough, I used to tell my wife that her high blood pressure, headaches, and probably backache must be due to our conflicts. However, I believed that since I was aware of my inner feelings and had trained myself to cope well under stress, I would not be a victim of tension-related illness. I felt a little relieved when I read a letter to Dr. Sarno from a clinical psychologist who had suffered from back pain and sciatica and, in spite of his expertise in psychology, had accepted the physical reasons for his pain.

My father suffered his share of debilitating back pain in his thirties. He has also experienced acne, TMJ, and hay fever, all of which I had as well. All my brothers have had back pain at one time or another—even the brother who is only sixteen years old. How much of that pain is due to tension and how much is genetics is hard to say. It is probably a combination of both.

My personal history is by no means unique. It illustrates how everyday life circumstances can be sources of tension and lead to pain and other physical symptoms. Also, Physical manifestations of tension can be experienced at any stage of life and are a normal reaction to life's many stressful circumstances. The good news is that we can challenge and overcome many of these physical manifestation of tension.

POSITIVE THINKING

Throughout my months of pain and disability I tried to be positive and hope that when and if I recovered I would do my best to become a healthy, strong person. Thanks to Dr. Sarno and the grace of God, I not only recovered from back pain but was relieved of many other physical manifestations of tension as well—and no longer suffer from hay fever or need my reading glasses.

THE MIND/BODY BENEFITS

More important, I learned more about the mind/body connection and its vital role in causing illness and healing. So far, I've experienced the following benefits as a result:

- Requiring fewer doctor visits, tests, and procedures
- Facing less chance for improper diagnoses and treatments
- Saving hours at doctors offices and clinics
- Being spared the uncertainties and frustrations of conflicting diagnoses
- Rarely taking any medications

- Saving on medical expenses
- Harnessing my mind's power and abilities to combat pain
- Utilizing my body's natural healing system
- Feeling a greater sense of confidence in dealing with health problems
- Enjoying better health, and a more pleasurable life because of it.

I have also learned to say no, especially to those closest to me. Whenever my conscientious side bothers me, I remind myself of all the agony and disability I suffered because I was trying to please everyone close to me. I still try to be as accommodating as possible, but I am far more aware of my limitations, and I expect—and when necessary demand—to be treated with respect and understanding.

I will appreciate these benefits for the rest of my life. Stress and tension are an integral part of our daily lives and at any age we may face stressful situations that can affect our health; but knowledge of the mind/body connection can indeed help us overcome the physical symptoms more quickly and easily. In the next chapter I will discuss in detail the nine-step rapid recovery plan and how you can become pain-free too.

6

THE NINE-STEP RAPID RECOVERY PLAN

*T*hus far you have learned:

- The correct diagnosis for most chronic back, neck, and hand pain
- The physiological changes that cause the pain
- How the pain becomes chronic
- How this knowledge can help you recover
- How I was able to recover rapidly using simple yet highly effective techniques

In this chapter you will learn:

- How the recovery plan has helped others recover rapidly
- How you can apply it to your condition
- How to design your own rapid recovery plan

You might be wondering whether you too can recover just as fast.[1] Of course, I would not be surprised if you are one of the many men and women who begin to improve as they learn this information. Case in point: A family friend called me a few weeks ago. She had suffered from six months of recurrent back and leg pain. She was frustrated with her medical treatment and had shown very little improvement.

As I talked to her on the telephone, she began to apply my techniques and experienced immediate improvements. I told her that one of the ways you can tell chronic back pain is caused by tension is that patients begin to get better as they become excited about the possibility of rapid recovery. This feeling of hope and excitement increases blood flow to their muscles, and they improve. She commented, "That's so true! I am already getting better. I am walking around as we speak and feeling less pain!" She recovered within forty-eight hours.

In fact, you are even more likely than she was to improve quickly and recover rapidly. After all, when you read a book at your own pace and focus on the material presented, it is easier to absorb the information and understand it. So it is very likely that, as your fear of pain was reduced due to the information you just learned, you found yourself sitting in one position a little longer than usual or testing your ability to move a little more. These are what I call quick confidence-building improvements.

This chapter is designed to walk you through the nine-step rapid recovery plan. You will not only learn more about these techniques and why they are so powerful, but also be able to practice each technique after it is explained. This practice will prepare you for the last section of this chapter, which helps you design your own rapid recovery plan, to make your recovery even faster and easier.

---

[1] This section is meant to provide a practical guide for those suffering from chronic or recurring back pain that is not caused by a serious medical condition. Always consult a physician to eliminate the possibility of a serious condition such as cancer, infection, or bone disease.

CASES OF RAPID RECOVERY

As mentioned earlier, many of the techniques you are about to learn use communication modes best understood by the subconscious mind, as well as other mental techniques that rapidly reverse the physical manifestations of tension. These simple yet highly effective techniques can produce amazing results, as the following cases demonstrate.

Rapid Recovery from Back and Leg Pain

One case that demonstrates the power of these techniques is that of Barbara.[2] A thirty-three-year-old teacher and mother of two, Barbara had suffered from back pain and left-leg pain for a year and was diagnosed with a bulging disc at the L4-5 vertebrae. She began to have back pain after completing an important project at work. She had received conventional treatments as well as chiropractic manipulation. When I met her she was off work on disability for the second time in a year.

Barbara sat very uncomfortably as we spoke and had to get up and walk around a few times to alleviate her pain. She was unable to bend at all or to sit for more than twenty minutes. She could only walk normally for about ten minutes at a time, after which her left leg became stiff and she began to limp. She had difficulty standing in one place for more than five minutes and was in constant pain. She was afraid of going to bed at night because of the severity of the pain in the morning, and the anti-inflammatory medication her doctor had prescribed was not relieving her pain anymore either.

She was a stark reminder of what I had suffered. I shared with her my experiences with chronic back and leg pain. I also explained about TMS and how I was able to recover so rapidly from this disabling condition. Then I helped her design a recovery plan like mine.

---

[2] Names of individuals, and in some cases personal information, have been altered to protect their privacy.

I asked Barbara to tell herself before going to sleep—using strong emotions and the proper physical reinforcements, such as a serious expression on her face and clenched fists—that she was not going to hurt anymore. I asked her to visualize herself carrying out her activities free of pain, and to visualize these scenes as vividly as possible, in color and with sounds and smells she associated with success and feeling great.

I also advised her to stop fearing pain and to ignore or push against it in careful, gradual, planned steps.[3] We also set some short-term and long-term goals. For the first day her goal was to try to bend twenty degrees, to sit for thirty minutes, to stand comfortably for longer than five minutes, and to walk for more than twelve minutes. She was to increase the time for each activity or position every day, and since she loved coffee-flavored Häagen-Dazs ice cream, we set that as her reward.

For her long-term goals she chose being absolutely pain-free while sitting on the floor, in seven days, and being able to carry her four-year-old daughter, the lighter of her two children, in fourteen days.

Although my explanation that tension was the main cause of her back and leg pain had made some sense to her, she was still skeptical. She also was not sure whether she would improve as rapidly as I had merely from following such simple and easy-to-apply steps. I told her that, as with any new concept or habit, it would take a few days or weeks for pain-free activity to be completely accepted by her mind and to become second nature. I advised her simply to put these strategies into practice and give her mind a few days to accept them. She was not familiar with

---

[3] As most people with chronic back pain know, on many occasions, such as when seeing a doctor or therapist, back patients have to ignore or push against their pain anyway. They end up sitting, standing, or maintaining other uncomfortable positions for longer periods than usual, and they have to tolerate the pain and discomfort. I remember many occasions when I returned home with more pain after going to the doctor or for therapy. Here we are taking control of the pain by not being afraid of it and gradually overcoming it.

Pavlov's experiments or conditioning and had not read much on psychology; however, as I was leaving she said, "I am still not convinced, but I will give it a try."

I called her the next day. Her husband answered the telephone. He was excited and extremely happy about his wife's improvement. "I finally got some sleep last night!" he told me. Apparently due to his wife's pain and discomfort, he had not been getting much sleep. Barbara was also overjoyed and amazed at her rapid recovery and told me that she had improved overnight. She slept better and woke up with much less pain. She could get out of bed faster, and her leg did not hurt as much. She said that certain leg positions that had hurt just a day earlier, and which she expected to hurt that day, did not. She was fighting back the pain and stiffness by moving around faster and with more vigor. She was able to bend about ten degrees and to sit for thirty minutes, and she was in much better condition than she had been the day before. She was also giving herself the ice cream reward we had discussed.

"Going in one day from being so disabled to make such a quick recovery is hard to believe!" Barbara exclaimed. She was afraid the pain might return at any time. I explained to her that this fear is a natural reaction to rapid change; but by keeping a daily record of her achievements, reviewing them, and keeping her goals in mind, she could build her confidence, remain motivated, and succeed in overcoming her fears and doubts, just as I had done.

I gave her a breathing exercise to help her relax, advised her to try to do more enjoyable things, such as taking time to really savor her ice cream reward, and to laugh more. I also asked her to read the letters patients had written to Dr. Sarno reprinted in the appendix to *Healing Back Pain,* which she had bought the day before.

I kept in touch with her by phone and she continued to improve, despite catching the flu, which forced her to stay in bed for about three days. When I met Barbara six days after my initial visit, she appeared quite relaxed and comfortable. She sat on the sofa as we spoke and told me that she was 90 percent pain-free. She had felt chest pains on the third day of her recovery but knew it was due to tension, and the pain subsided on its own. She could bend ninety degrees without feeling pain, walk long distances, stand for a long time, and sleep comfortably. She also sat on the floor, one of the goals she had set for herself.

Barbara told me that she felt young again. Her children were excited about her improvements and how she was doing things she could not have done just a few days earlier. She experienced pain when she sneezed, but told me that even though she expected to, she did not feel pain when she coughed. I told her to keep coughing and try to sneeze out the pain. I explained to her that for the next few weeks certain physical and emotional situations might cause pain, but that as she challenged those situations she would be able to eliminate pain faster and eventually become pain-free.

I explained to her about the mental exercises such as focusing and relaxation, and advised her to begin working out with weights, and to keep her goals in mind and record her progress daily for the next month in order to make this new habit of a pain-free body a firm and strong one.

Two days after this meeting, only eight days after she began her recovery and six days ahead of her goal schedule, she was able to carry her daughter. She loved the change in her life. She also told me she no longer had to think about where to sit or lie down. She was able to move freely, and she enjoyed her new freedom.

I explained to her that as she returned to work and her previous routine, there would be times in the first few weeks when she might feel pain due to tension or conditioning. But as long as she followed the steps we had discussed and kept a positive and determined attitude, she would be fine. She understood that her efforts to be the perfect wife, good employee, and supermom were the cause of her tension.

Herniated Disc

Joseph had suffered from three years of back and leg pain. It began a week after he moved his electrical equipment company to a larger facility. While building a shelf there, he twisted and felt pain in his back. Later he woke up with more pain in his back, radiating down his right leg. Despite many sessions of physical therapy and two cortisone shots, he continued to have pain. He had difficulty standing or sitting in one place for more than a few minutes. He also found it difficult to carry his five-year-old daughter.

Finally, a neurologist ordered an MRI of Joseph's back. The MRI showed a herniated disc at the L4-L5 vertebrae. Joseph was told that he needed surgery. He was a well-built, active man and in good health prior to his back pain. The prospect of surgery really bothered him.

He had heard about my seminars on back pain through friends, and he called me to arrange for a meeting. I shared with him the many studies that demonstrate the lack of correlation between a herniated disc and back pain, and the ineffectiveness of surgery. I explained to him about TMS and the conditioned response. He listened intently but seemed skeptical. However, as I explained to him the characteristics of TMS and how the pain moves around, his face lit up.

"So that's what it is!" he exclaimed. "When I put an ice pack on my foot the pain moves to my calf, and when I put a second ice pack on my calf, it moves to my thigh. Just last week I told my wife that I needed a third ice pack to put on my thigh." I was glad to see how an explanation of TMS had helped him make sense of his condition.

Then I helped him design his own rapid recovery plan. He wanted to be able to stand in one place for five minutes for the first day and to increase the time to thirty minutes by the end of the week. For his ultimate goal he wanted to carry his daughter after one week and to run five miles after two weeks.

"Don't you think running five miles is a bit too much, since you are not running at all right now?" I asked him.

"You said I need to set an ultimate goal that makes me excited about recovery. Well, running five miles is what makes me excited about recovery," he answered.

"If that's the case, go for it. But if you end up running two miles that's still something to be excited about," I told him.

At the end of our meeting he asked, "But what about the herniated disc in my back?" I reviewed the research with him once more and told him that it was his decision how he wanted to proceed. He told me he was going to give the recovery plan a try.

One week later I called him. He had recovered rapidly. Standing and sitting in one position was quite easy now. He was carrying his daughter without difficulty and running about thirty minutes every other day. He felt some pain but was no longer afraid of it or worried about it. He was not able to run five miles after two weeks, but he continued to run about thirty minutes three to four times a week, to give back rides to his daughter, and to take care of the new member of his family, a baby boy.

Chronic Pain Due to an Automobile Accident

And then there was John. He was a twenty-nine-year-old computer scientist and businessman who had been in two serious car accidents in six years. The first time he was broadsided by a truck and taken to the hospital unconscious. He woke up later feeling pain all over and continued to have pain and muscle spasms from his left shoulder down to his left leg. Therapy and medication helped but did not eliminate the pain. To make matters worse, six years later he was rear-ended on the freeway by a car traveling thirty miles per hour faster than his.

John suffered from severe sciatica in his left leg, piriformis syndrome, and chronic pain from his neck to his lower back. He also experienced pain and numbness in both forearms and hands at night and when he held them in a raised position, such as when holding a telephone receiver. His orthopedically designed bed was not much help, and he had to sleep on the floor. This situation was emotionally painful for him, as he was newly married and his bride found sleeping on the floor quite uncomfortable.

I explained TMS and the recovery plan to him, and since he was a self-motivated, goal-oriented person, I let him design his own recovery plan. Shortly after our meeting he began sleeping on the sofa, and in less than two weeks he was sleeping on his bed without experiencing any pain or discomfort. John's wife, mother, other relatives, and friends were amazed at his rapid improvement. He rewarded himself by taking his wife out to dinner.

Thereafter, he experienced only mild and occasional bouts of back pain, which he was able to eliminate on command; however, the numbness in his forearms and hands had not improved, especially on the right side. He had had two operations on his right wrist to help relieve pressure in the past, and he worried that he might need more surgery. I told him that considering his triumph over pain in his back, he should seriously consider challenging the numbness in his forearms and hands as well. Then I explained to him one of the techniques I had used that was quite effective: scaring the pain away!

I used to hit myself on my thighs or other parts of my body that hurt to prove to my mind that my body was healthy, and I was no longer afraid of pain. I had also threatened my subconscious that if it did not stop the pain in my back or leg, I would give it such a pain that the pain caused by tension would fade in comparison. Of course, I followed up by pushing as hard as I could against the pain—by getting into the positions and doing the activities that caused pain. This approach had worked very well. So I advised John to give this strategy a try, too.

When I met John one week later, he said his forearm and hand had improved tremendously. Any time he felt pain or numbness, he grasped his right forearm firmly and told his inner child he would do worse if it did not stop the pain. I was glad to see that this technique worked for him and that he was able to avoid another operation.

I should add here that whiplash-associated disorders from a car accident are also related to tension. That is why most people feel neck pain and headaches the day following an accident. A test manager who had suffered from whiplash for three weeks recovered rapidly following my plan (please read his letter in Appendix B). The McGill University study discussed in the introduction found that nine out of ten patients recovered from whiplash if left alone.[4] Thus, ignoring the pain made it go away.

Neck and Arm Pain

Adam, a forty-year-old electrical engineer, was a perfectionist overachiever with a doctorate in electrical engineering from Stanford University. He was involved in research as well as teaching at two University of California campuses.

Adam suffered for one and a half years from chronic pain in his neck and right shoulder, and pain and numbness in his right arm and two fingers. He had difficulty sitting and typing on the computer for more than fifteen minutes, a circumstance that was making him consider major changes in his career. He was seen by a general practitioner, two chiropractors, and eventually by a neurosurgeon at a prestigious university hospital. The neurosurgeon had recommended neck surgery based on the MRI findings. Three bulging discs were found, the worst of which was at the C6-7 vertebrae.

He was advised to restrict his activity to avoid further damage to his neck. He had been an avid athlete all his life and missed his rigorous exercise regimen, which included swimming, jogging, gymnastics, soccer, and tennis.

Adam told me that the pain began one night while he was working on the computer, and was so severe that he went to the emergency room. As we talked more, it was clear that he was upset over a number of issues related to his job. Since he had been very efficient in completing various projects ahead of schedule, he was expected to carry most of the workload while some of his coworkers took it easy.

---

[4] Spitzer, Walter O., et al., "Scientific Monograph of the Quebec Task Force on Whiplash-Associated Disorders," *Spine* 20 (1995): 34S–39S.

Adam understood TMS and what he needed t
of the pain. His goals for the first day included be
longer and to type on the computer for twenty minutes, and for
seven days later, being able to walk on his hands! He loved
walking on his hands, but he had been warned about its
detrimental effects on his neck. He was happy and excited about
not needing a surgery. As he was leaving, he told me that he had
already started telling himself that he was not going to hurt
anymore; he said he felt 90 percent less pain.

The next day he was able to type on the computer for an
entire hour without any difficulty, and he no longer experienced
sharp pains in his neck and arm. One week later he was able to
walk on his hands as planned. He recovered quickly, experiencing
occasional mild pain in his neck, and one month after he walked
on his hands again he put an end to his life as a bachelor and
married the "perfect" wife.

Interestingly enough, when Adam showed his neurosurgeon
some of the medical articles I had given him on the failures of
surgery and the lack of correlation between disc abnormalities and
pain, the surgeon shrugged his shoulders and told Adam,
"Whatever works for you!" Just a few days earlier the same
neurosurgeon had recommended neck surgery based on MRI
results, and now he did not seem to think surgery was
important—more evidence that it is crucial to be an informed
patient.

Knee Pain

There was also Stephen, an obstetrician/gynecologist who
woke up one morning to severe pain in his right knee—pain so
severe that he needed a cane to walk, and still had great difficulty
getting around and climbing stairs. Once I explained to him about
TMS and the nine-step recovery plan, he improved rapidly. I saw
him the next day walking, as he put it, "vigorously," with only a
slight limp. He experienced very little difficulty after that, and
recovered completely shortly afterward.

Carpal Tunnel Syndrome

This recovery plan has also helped several people with symptoms of chronic pain and numbness in their hands and arms. One of them was Daniel, a facility manager who had been diagnosed with carpal tunnel syndrome. His left hand had been operated on, and he was scheduled for an operation on his right hand as well. He too recovered rapidly and avoided surgery on his right hand. I will discuss his case in detail when I explain more about the recovery plan.

Foot Pain

Once I was discussing the benefits of exercise with Bill, the president of a computer company. He sighed and said, "Yeah! When I was younger, I was involved in all kinds of sports, and even won a few trophies. But for the past three years I have had this pain in my feet that has limited my activities considerably. I guess I am getting old."

He did not look too old to me, so I asked about his age.

"I'll be fifty in thirteen years!"

Bill had developed foot pain after playing basketball three years earlier. He attributed the injury to his being out of shape and not wearing suitable shoes for playing basketball. He was limited to standing and walking for about fifteen minutes at a time. He had tried many treatments and remedies without success, and had stopped playing basketball and participating in other sports activities because of his condition.

I explained briefly about my experience, told him that he would probably recover very quickly, and offered to do a presentation at his company. I had met Bill before, and I knew that he was a very determined and persistent individual. Also, as the president of the company, he was in control of his life to a greater degree than most people are. This combination of having a strong personality and being in control is very helpful in speeding up recovery.

Bill attended my presentation, and although not fully convinced, he decided to try my techniques. As I had suspected, he recovered within twenty-four hours and went on to play basketball and even soccer.

Another case of foot pain was Andrew. He was a friend of mine and the cofounder of an electronics company, suffered from heel pain for a few months. X-rays revealed calcium deposits in his heel. His doctor advised him to try physical therapy first and recommended surgery if there was no improvement. However, the doctor told Andrew that surgery does not have a high success rate in such cases. Andrew also recovered rapidly following the rapid recovery plan. You may read about his recovery in Appendix B.

Chronic Bronchitis

I received a call from Susan, an engineering professor who had been suffering for seven years from chronic bronchitis. She had been given a wide range of diagnoses and treatments, but nothing had worked. She coughed constantly. In the course of our conversation she had to stop several times, and she coughed so much that her whole face turned red.

This incessant coughing had made Susan's life miserable. She was using a cortisone inhaler to keep the coughing under control. She told me that sometimes in the middle of a lecture she had to leave the classroom because of her cough. She had noticed that she did not cough when focused on a task or when exercising. However, she coughed afterward. The dust from the blackboard made her cough, although she was not allergic to it prior to her bronchitis. She had tried transcendental meditation, and it had helped a little.

Since she had had this condition for seven years, I suspected she had a clue to its real cause. So I asked her, "What do you think is the cause of your chronic cough?"

"Do you want me to tell you what doctors have told me?"

I said, "No. I want to know what you think is the cause."

"I feel like I am carrying the whole world on my shoulders, and that is what is causing my cough!" she responded.

Well, it did not take much explaining on my part to help her realize that tension was the cause of her cough. I helped Susan design her own rapid recovery plan. She was going to give herself a piece of chocolate if she did not cough for ten minutes for the first day. She was to increase the time every day until she was cough-free.

And did it work! The first day she did not cough for an entire hour, and she continued to improve as planned. However, on the day her son was taking the dental school entrance exam she coughed more than before. She realized that even though she did not think she felt especially anxious about the exam, in fact it was creating enough anxiety and tension to make her cough. Susan continued on the plan and recovered completely. She recovered so well that she was no longer allergic to the blackboard dust, either.

I wondered why she had developed a cough in response to tension. Unlike others whose backs or hands are the focus of their work, as a professor she used her voice on the job. So tension manifested itself in a way that affected her voice, as a chronic cough!

Hereditary Hemorrhagic Telangiectasia

Once I called Victor, a design manager acquaintance of mine, to ask him a question. He sounded very ill on the phone. I asked him whether he had a cold.

He said, "No. I have a condition called hereditary hemorrhagic telangiectasia, or HHT for short. It is a hereditary and chronic condition that causes nosebleeds. I have had it for ten years and have tried everything from laser surgery to medications, but nothing has worked." He told me that he usually bled at night, in his sleep, and first thing in the morning. He rarely bled at work. "Aha!" I thought—a possible case of TMS equivalent.

I set a time to meet with him. He was late due to excessive bleeding right before our meeting. He told me that most people with this condition experience bleeding after puberty and continue to have problems throughout their lives. His grandfather had to receive transfusions because he lost so much blood, and he eventually died from excessive bleeding. Victor was allergic to tea, coffee, and chocolate. If he had even a little bit of these, his nose bled. He had recently attended a national conference on HHT. Although many issues related to the cause and treatment of HHT were discussed, tension was never considered as a factor.

Considering that the bleeding began after puberty, when most teens experience a lot of tension, and that Victor bled at night and early in the morning, I surmised that the bleeding was his body's way of manifesting tension. When I explained to him that TMS seemed likely to be involved, he agreed completely. In fact, he had noticed that when he was under stress, he experienced more serious bleeding.

Victor was ready to try the techniques. He was bleeding three times a day at the time. He also bled when he bent down. So we set the goal of reducing bleeding to twice a day, with ice cream as his reward. He was to bend down and not bleed after one week.

I called him two days later to find out that he had not bled at all and was doing great. Later he had some minor bleeding, but through applying stress-reduction techniques and balancing his responsibilities, he eventually had very few problems. He was able to bend without bleeding after one week, and he even drank coffee and ate chocolate with no aftereffects.

I have worked with many others who suffered TMS or TMS-equivalent symptoms. People who have applied these strategies have seen rapid improvement in their conditions, whether they had been suffering from back, neck, shoulder, or knee pain; numbness in their arms and hands; sciatica; chest pain; or some combination of these. Of course, all these people had been examined by physicians. Doctors either had given these patients conventional diagnoses and treatments for chronic back, leg, or knee pain, or else, in the case of chest pain, had ruled out organic causes.

I would consider it absolutely irresponsible and unethical to advise others about a medical condition without the benefit of a diagnosis by a qualified health care professional. Pain and numbness may be due to a tumor, diabetes, an infection, or some other disease or disorder, which if not treated in time could have dire consequences. For this reason, I have shared my experiences only with people who have already been medically examined.

One of the observations I have made from working with others is that you do not need to know much about psychology or to be absolutely convinced that your pain is caused by tension (at least in the short run) to recover. As long as you are truly motivated to take conscious charge of your condition and no longer accept being a helpless victim of pain, you can expect to recover rapidly by following the recovery plan.

As demonstrated, my nine-step recovery plan is simple, safe, easy to follow, and quite effective. It has produced rapid results for those who have seriously applied its techniques. The plan takes little time to do and has no negative side effects. In fact, those who have benefited from it have experienced many positive side effects, such as feeling youthful and having more vigor and energy, in addition to gaining a better, happier, and much more hopeful outlook on life. People who have followed the plan feel empowered to realize the potential they possess to bring about rapid changes for the better in their lives.

The purpose of most of the techniques in my nine-step recovery plan is not only to help you communicate effectively with your subconscious mind and motivate it to follow your commands, but also to let it know that you are in charge by helping you take conscious control of your thoughts and actions. The more you get away from the automatic (subconscious) mode of carrying out daily activities such as breathing, eating, and driving, the sooner you may expect to recover. Pay more attention to how you perform routine tasks. Concentrate on how you breathe, eat, or drive to make your subconscious mind more receptive to your command.

Another important advantage of these techniques is that they can benefit you for life. For there may be times when commanding the subconscious mind may not make it stop the pain or some other tension-related symptom; however, these strategies can always come to your aid in reducing or eliminating symptoms of TMS.

As you may recall, at one point my subconscious mind did not respond to my commands to stop my hay fever, and I kept on sneezing. But when I talked to it before sleep, visualized, set my goal of no sneezing, and promised ice cream as my reward, it responded quickly, and by the following day I was able to stop the allergic response.

These techniques can even help you eliminate warts. Once I developed a wart on my left hand two days after an incident that really made me upset. Using visualization, goal-setting, and the other techniques discussed here, I was able to eliminate the wart in six days. I showed my wife how the wart gradually dried up, shriveled, and went away. This experience was another wonderful confirmation of how effective these techniques can be.

In the pages that follow I have explained the wisdom behind these techniques and their benefits. When appropriate, action items are set out that will help you practice the techniques and facilitate your recovery. At the end of this chapter these action items are incorporated into an easy-to-follow action plan. There is also a progress chart that will help you record and celebrate your daily accomplishments.

It is important that you take your recovery one step at a time, and consider it an enjoyable and relaxing process. Keep in mind that as with other matters related to the mind, such as learning and problem solving, the more relaxed you are and the more you enjoy the process, the faster you can get the job done (I will expound more on this point in the step on mental exercises).

As mentioned earlier, the same way that we can prevent ourselves from crying when our eyes fill with tears due to sadness—an emotion leading to physiological change—we have the ability to increase blood flow to the affected muscles, nerves, tendons, and ligaments, and relieve the resulting pain or numbness. It is simply a matter of believing that you can and taking the necessary steps with the intention of getting well. And why not? Thousands have been able to recover from this chronic painful condition, and so can you.

Besides, here you will not only learn the importance of each technique and how it works, but you will also have an opportunity to practice each one before designing your rapid recovery plan. I have provided you with an easy action item for each technique so that you can develop a better understanding of how to apply the techniques as well as practice them for faster results. At the end of this section, I will take you step by step through the techniques and help you design your personal rapid recovery plan.

THE NINE-STEP RAPID RECOVERY PLAN

Now here is the nine-step rapid recovery plan:

1. **MOTIVATION**
2. **POSITIVE THINKING**
3. **MENTAL EXERCISES**
4. **GOAL-SETTING**
5. **REWARD AND PUNISHMENT**
6. **DAILY RECORD**
7. **EXERCISE**
8. **SELF-DISCIPLINE**
9. **DESENSITIZATION AND POSITIVE ASSOCIATION**

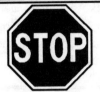

Now I want you to take a moment and do something very simple that will maximize the benefits you will get from this recovery plan. I want you to close your eyes, focus, and create the intention in your heart and in your mind that every action you take now will help you recover rapidly. You might want to say to yourself,

"Every step I take from now on will help me to recover faster and faster."

Make a fist and say these words with a serious expression on your face. Make this statement to yourself several times with strong feelings and determination.

1. Motivation

Motivation is the key to taking action and a key ingredient for success in any endeavor. Olympic athletes and high achievers know how important it is to become motivated and stay motivated in order to achieve their goals. To recover rapidly, you too need to be truly motivated to get rid of the pain and live a healthy, active life.

But how do you become motivated? The answer lies within you! The more reasons you have for rapid recovery, the more likely it is for you to become motivated, apply the techniques, and regain your health. The two motivating reasons for our actions are avoiding pain and gaining pleasure. In order to help you attach a lot of emotional pain to back and neck pain and disability, and a lot of pleasure to living pain-free and healthy, I have devised the following exercise for you.

This exercise will help you attach a lot of pain to living with recurrent and chronic pain, so that you make every effort to avoid living with pain and take action to get well. If you are truly motivated to take action and recover, you may skip this exercise and complete the one that focuses on the benefits and pleasures you gain by recovering rapidly.

ACTION ITEM

1. **Take a moment and think about at least five opportunities you missed due to chronic pain.**
2. **Now consider five opportunities or activities you are unable to benefit from now and will be prevented from enjoying in the future because of chronic pain.**
3. **Make yourself feel the emotional pain associated with these lost opportunities and get mad at the pain. Decide now that you will put an end to this pain!**
4. **Now, to increase the pleasure associated with recovery, think of at least five wonderful benefits and pleasures you will enjoy by making a rapid recovery and living pain-free.**

A motivation list can help you stay focused and give you the determination you need throughout the recovery period. It will make you realize the true impact this painful condition has on your life and help you stay focused on the wonderful benefits you will gain by recovering. I believe you will find that the prospect of getting rid of the pain, regaining your health, not having to ask others for help, and enjoying a good night's sleep is motivation enough. But how about the motivation that thoughts of your loved ones, your career, and your plans for the future can provide?

Now for increasing the pleasure you associated with rapid recovery do the following exercise:

ACTION ITEM
1. Take a moment and think about five activities you will participate in the next seven days as you recover. Imagine how good you will feel as you do them.
2. Now consider five activities you will participate in one month from now as a healthy, pain-free person. Notice how wonderful it feels to be pain-free and active.
3. Now extend the following exercise to six months from now, imagine how good you will feel, and record those feelings in your mind.

---

2. Positive Thinking

As mentioned earlier, one of the best ways to communicate with the subconscious mind is through strong emotions and the images associated with them. Also, since TMS is caused by repressed anger and other negative emotions, it is very important to maintain a hopeful, positive attitude while challenging it; you must approach your recovery with the intention that everything you do will take you a step closer to your complete recovery. [5]

Be calm and confident and apply these strategies with positive expectations. In this step you are going to use strong positive emotions and associated images to bring about desired change for a pain-free body. Before sleep is usually the time when the subconscious mind is most receptive to our conscious commands.

---

[5] Here positive thinking includes positive self-talk, positive attitude, and positive emotions and feelings.

ACTION ITEM

Close your eyes, take a deep breath, clench your fists, concentrate, and say to yourself,

"I am not going to hurt anymore. I will certainly win my battle against pain."

Say this at least five times, with a positive, determined attitude and a serious expression on your face. Feel strong, powerful, and unstoppable.

Continue to repeat this statement to yourself when you wake up and throughout the day. When you do this during the day, stand erect and tall (if you can).

Act tough by putting more energy into whatever you do. Show your subconscious mind that you are in charge now. This attitude is what I call "body over mind." You must approach your recovery with a positive, determined attitude, to show your subconscious that you are confident that it will obey your commands and make the necessary changes. This approach means resolving that, no matter how long you have had this pain and how severe your level of disability is, God willing, you are going to overcome your pain. Think of others who were able to succeed in this challenge and realize that you have the potential, as all humans do, to conquer your pain.

People who have tried my methods have found this step extremely effective. In fact, many people have told me that after repeating this statement, before going to sleep, they have noticed overnight improvement in their level of pain and numbness, whether they were suffering from back and leg pain or pain and numbness in their hands. This is the first step to realizing that they exert some control over their pain and that they can use their minds and innate abilities to reduce pain and to recover.

In one such case, during an inspection I learned that Daniel, a facility manager in his early forties, had been diagnosed with carpal tunnel syndrome. He had been experiencing pain and numbness in both hands for eight months. His left hand had been operated on, but his condition had not improved. He was scheduled for an operation on his right hand when we met.

He was clearly distressed and frustrated by the ineffectiveness of the treatments he had received so far and by the inability of the specialists to answer his questions about his condition. I described my experience with back pain and the pain and numbness in my forearms and hands. I suggested that he get mad at the pain and say to himself, "I am not going to hurt anymore," every night before going to sleep. I also suggested that he visualize himself being pain-free and healthy.

The following week I stopped by to give Daniel a copy of *Healing Back Pain* and ask about his hands. He said he had been following my suggestion every night, and that in the mornings his hands had been fine, but later in the day, when he began to worry about the pain, the tingling and numbness returned. However, there had been times during the day when he had been pain-free for an hour or two.

I met Daniel again two weeks later. By then he had read Dr. Sarno's book and said he had developed a better understanding of TMS. He had also realized how much anger and frustration he had been keeping inside, and the stress he felt from his efforts to be the perfect employee. The pain and numbness in his hands had begun after he started working on a project that required a great deal of manual work, a project that would have cost the company three times more if a contractor had done it. However, being a model employee, he accepted his employer's request to undertake the project in addition to his other responsibilities. At that point, he began to experience pain and numbness in his hands.[6]

Daniel told me that he still experienced some numbness. However, he had been pain-free and had done some plumbing work, which he could not do before. The swelling of his hands had improved so much that he could take his wedding ring off his finger when he woke up in the morning; later he canceled the second surgery. Interestingly enough, a few days into his recovery he woke up one morning with back pain. Since he knew that tension-related pain

---

[6] In *The Mindbody Prescription* Dr. Sarno mentions carpal tunnel syndrome as another manifestation of TMS (New York, N.Y.: Warner Books, 1998), pp. 94–95.

moves around, he continued to tell the pain to go away, and after about ten minutes the pain subsided. Needless to say, he was quite happy and excited about his new discovery.

Now that you know how powerful and effective this technique is, I want you to practice it one more time. Close your eyes, take a deep breath, clench your fists, concentrate, and tell yourself, "I am not going to hurt anymore." Do not read another word until you have repeated this statement at least five times.

Seriously practice this technique, and keep a positive, confident attitude about your recovery. Certainly you may experience a relapse due to tension, as I did, you may find that you do not improve as fast as you had hoped; but you should keep thinking, acting, and moving positively and keep telling yourself that you will overcome the pain. View any setback as another challenge to be met and won.

3. Mental Exercises

Since TMS is caused by the subconscious mind, it is imperative to apply the following mental exercises to the best of your abilities. However, keep in mind that in contrast to physical matters—where the harder you apply yourself the sooner you see results—matters of the mind are accomplished much more easily and rapidly when we relax and enjoy the process.

We all have had the experience of trying hard to remember a name or telephone number with no success. It seems the harder we try and the more anxious we become, the less likely it is that we will recall the information. However, later on when we relax, or during some unrelated activity, such as driving or grocery shopping, the name or number suddenly pops up in our minds.

Being relaxed not only helps our minds recall information faster and more easily, but also facilitates the learning process. Have you noticed how much better you learn when an instructor teaches in a relaxed environment and presents the information with a lot of visual aids and humor? In other words, when we are relaxed and enjoy ourselves, our minds learn, memorize, analyze, remember, and solve problems with much greater efficiency. So, as you do the following mental exercises, concentrate and put in the necessary effort, but remember to relax and enjoy yourself as well.

I have used the following mental exercises for many years as a result of my studies in psychology and my experience with the subconscious mind. These exercises—imagery and visualization, focusing, and relaxation—will provide you with some basic tools to keep your mind in tune and help you use its various capabilities, such as its power of imagination, to combat chronic pain and improve your overall health.

Imagery and Visualization. As you have already seen, since the mind thinks in pictures, presenting it with the right images is a very effective means of communicating with it and can speed up the recovery process amazingly. Moviemakers and advertisers are well aware of the powerful effects of images on our minds and use images very effectively. In this exercise you will be making your own mental movies. You are going to be the producer, the director, and the actor—or should I say—the hero.

Before I discuss this technique, however, I would like to put you through an exercise commonly used to demonstrate the effects of mental images on our bodies. Read the following, then close your eyes and imagine doing it.

> *You are standing in your kitchen in front of a cutting board. Next to it is a good sharp knife. Take a few moments to imagine the kitchen: the color of the countertops, the appliances, the cupboards, the windows, and so on. Also notice*

> *any kitchen smells or sounds—the running of a*
> *dishwasher or the hum of a refrigerator.*
>
> *Now imagine that on the board sits a*
> *plump, fresh, juicy lemon. In your mind, hold*
> *the lemon in one hand, feeling its weight and*
> *texture. Then place it back on the board and*
> *carefully cut it in half with the knife. Feel the*
> *resistance to the knife and how it gives way as*
> *the lemon splits. Notice the pale yellow of the*
> *pulp, the whiteness of the inner peel, and see*
> *whether you have cut through a seed or two.*
> *Carefully cut one of the halves in two. See where*
> *a drop or two of juice pearled on the surface of*
> *one of the quarters. Imagine lifting this lemon*
> *wedge to your mouth, smelling the sharp fresh*
> *scent. Now bite into the sour, juicy pulp.* [7]

The above exercise causes most people to salivate—a physiological change. Although there was no actual lemon and the entire event took place in your imagination, your mind treated the experience as real and increased saliva secretion, which was the appropriate physical response. This example demonstrates two

---

[7] *Imagery: Learning to Use the Mind's Eye* by Dr. Martin Rossman as quoted in *Mind Body Medicine,* edited by Daniel Goleman and Joel Gurin (Yonkers, N.Y.: Consumer Reports Books, 1993), p. 295. Dr. Rossman is a clinical associate in the Department of Medicine at the University of California, San Francisco, and codirector of the Academy for Guided Imagery in Mill Valley, California. I highly recommend Dr. Martin Rossman's book, *Healing Yourself: A Step-by-Step Program to Better Health by Imagery* (New York: Pocket Books, 1987). In this book he describes treating thousands of patients for back pain, asthma, headaches, high blood pressure, palpitations, and allergies using imagery and visualization techniques. Imagery has also helped patients suffering disorders as diverse as endometriosis and recurrent infections to regain their health. Dr. Rossman has a series of self-help audio tapes that teach these techniques, available through Insight Publishing, P.O. Box 2070, Mill Valley, CA 94942; call (800) 726-2070.

very significant points: (1) our minds treat all images as real and create the appropriate physiological response to those images; (2) the images and thoughts that come into our minds daily, consciously or unconsciously, have certain effects on our bodies. As subtle as these effects might be on the conscious level, they can have positive or negative effects on our physiology. They can enhance our health or cause disease, depending on what images come to our minds and how much emotional impact is attached to them.

If images of an argument with your spouse or boss come to your mind repeatedly, these images could lead to physiological responses such as reduced blood flow to your back muscles and back pain.[8] Positive images, on the other hand, could have positive impacts on your health, such as an increased number of immune cells and better resistance to diseases.

Visualization is so effective that it has become an integral part of training programs for top athletes. In 1988 Dr. Shane Murphy, a sports psychologist, was assigned by the United States Olympic Committee to teach visualization to athletes. In fact, many top athletes, such as Jerry Rice of the San Francisco 49ers and Mary Lou Retton of the U.S. Olympic gymnastics team, visualize every move before the competition and boost their performances.[9]

This positive effect of visualization has also been proven effective among patients undergoing rehabilitation from heart attacks. "One group was given a typical physical exercise program; the other group was asked to perform the same program imaginally rather than physically. When the recovery rates of the two groups were compared, the imagery group was found to have

---

[8] I will give you a highly effective method for scrambling such negative thoughts in Chapter Seven. This simple, yet highly effective, visualization exercise can turn the images and feelings associated with a very upsetting experience to ones that make you laugh every time you think about it. It has worked wonders for me.

[9] Ornish, Dean, M.D., pp. 172–173. Visualization is an integral part of Dr. Ornish's program for reversing heart disease.

recovered much more quickly."[10] Using this technique can indeed help us utilize more of our inner abilities to meet life's challenges, such as back pain, and heal.[11]

Learning about and practicing imagery and visualization can have a dramatic impact on your health. Visualizing the appropriate images, sounds, and smells and combining these with strong positive emotions can facilitate your recovery from chronic back pain. This knowledge can also help you exert more control over the images that come to your mind and their impact on your health.

Since your mind has become conditioned to expect and cause pain when you are in certain positions or during certain activities, using your imagination to do the things that are usually painful and difficult, but without pain or discomfort, will make your mind accept the fact that those tasks can be done without pain. And since the subconscious takes over when you sleep, it is best to imagine doing those tasks without pain while you are calm and relaxed just before sleep. For faster results you can also do this as often as possible throughout the day. Just visualize yourself sitting, walking, and bending without feeling any pain. Imagine how free and wonderful it would feel to do all these activities comfortably. You can close your eyes, take a deep breath, and visualize yourself doing those tasks with great ease and pleasure right before actually doing them.

This is something that can be done as often as you want and takes very little time. The more you do it with positive feelings and a sense of triumph, the sooner your mind will accept that those tasks are supposed to be pain-free.

---

[10] Epstein, Gerald, M.D., *Healing Visualization: Creating Health Through Imagery* (New York: Bantam Books, 1989), p. 200. This is also a very valuable book on visualization.

[11] An active imagination can also help in eliminating warts, a TMS equivalent (*The Healing Brain* [New York: Simon & Shuster, 1987]), and enhance one's immune system in its fight against disease (*Prevention Magazine's 30-Day Immune Power Program* [Emmaus, Pa.: Rodale Press, 1992]).

ACTION ITEM

1. Take a moment and choose a symbol of power and strength. This can be yourself involved in an activity that makes you feel strong, or it can be your favorite athlete or movie action hero winning a competition or a fight. People have told me a wide range of these symbols, from a raging bull and ocean waves to the Bionic Woman and a race car.

2. Now close your eyes and imagine yourself for a few seconds actually doing that activity or being in the place of your symbol of power. Put a lot of feelings into it. Feel strong, powerful, and unstoppable. Change your posture to match those feelings. Do this at least five times. Really feel it.

3. Now close your eyes again and imagine doing your daily activities such as sitting, standing, or walking without pain. Imagine yourself doing them for hours at a time in complete ease, feeling triumphant over pain. Imagine that as you perform your daily activities you become that symbol of power and strength.

4. Practice the above action item at least five times. Make your images as colorful as you can and add sounds and movement to them. Do not worry if your images are not crystal clear. Just try to focus your mind on doing the activities.

It may take a few sessions of doing this exercise to see some improvement, but the more active your imagination is, the more feelings and sounds associated with triumph and victory you put into the exercise, the sooner you will see results. Try to see things as vividly as possible, in color and complete detail.

As I mention in the section on positive thinking, you can use visualization to create strong positive emotions that will help in facilitating your recovery. You can make yourself feel strong and powerful by seeing yourself as your favorite movie character or hero, defeating the pain warriors and winning back your health.

You can also imagine yourself as a tank and your pain as

brick walls. See yourself blasting through the walls of pain one by one triumphantly. Hear the sounds of the blasts and walls falling, and feel your strength increasing with each blast.

In another scenario, you can imagine that barriers of reinforced concrete are built around the areas of your back and neck where the pain is most severe. These barriers successfully keep any attack by the subconscious away from those areas, leaving you pain-free and relaxed. Find the images that are most effective for you.

When you do these visualizations, if you feel powerful and strong, are enthused and thrilled, or better yet get goose bumps, that is a good indication that you are really stirring up some strong positive emotions and feelings. This will in turn make your subconscious more receptive to your conscious desires and commands.

Focusing. This is another excellent means of training the subconscious to obey you. Focusing helps to concentrate all of your mind's attention and energy on one thought or action. It helps you to be in the present, stop feeling bad about the past, and quit worrying about the future; you can concentrate on whatever you happen to be doing at the time. Focusing is also a form of meditation. As mentioned earlier, since a preschooler wants to always be moving and be entertained, focusing on one word and staying in one position is not something the childlike subconscious likes. By doing so, you are teaching it to be patient and disciplined.

You can easily incorporate a focusing exercise into your daily routine. Since I do a lot of city driving, I focused on God's glory every time I had to wait at a stoplight. Of course, associated with this thought is the greatness of creation and God's great mercy, so this not only keeps my mind focused, but also leaves me filled with positive emotions and energy.

Making it a point to focus a few minutes, several times a day, on a particular word, such as *relax*, or *one*, will teach your mind to keep out all negative thoughts that interfere with the task at hand and to keep focused on doing the activity well.

ACTION ITEM
Choose a word that makes you relax or is associated with goodness in your life. Then focus your thoughts on it by saying it to yourself five times while keeping your eyes focused on a particular point—this helps train your mind as well as your body to stay focused. Gradually increase the number of sets you can do to five sets of five to ten repetitions. Do this exercise at least three times a day.

Each session takes less than sixty seconds to do. It not only helps focus your mind and improve your concentration, but it gives you a break from all the negative, tension-causing thoughts that come to your mind. You will notice that, like other skills, it takes a bit of practice. Your subconscious mind does not like this new change in your thinking pattern and will interrupt by distracting you. However, all you have to do is gently refocus your mind on that word and continue with your count.

Do not aim for perfect focus and concentration. Even those who have done this type of mental exercise for years tend to get distracted. Just remember that you are doing something good for yourself and what is important is that you put in the time and effort to do it. This shows your subconscious that you are serious about recovering from back pain.

Relaxation. There are a number of ways to achieve relaxation and release from tension. They range from deep belly breathing and progressive relaxation to meditation and autogenic exercises.

The following exercise involves tightening different muscle groups while taking a deep breath, holding your breath as much as possible, and letting go of the breath and muscle tension at the same time. It is quite easy and takes only a few minutes to do. By releasing stress and tension it provides you with more energy and vigor when you do it during the day, and a deep and restful sleep when you do it in bed the last thing at night.

1. Make sure you will not be disturbed.
2. Get into a comfortable position, lying down or sitting in a favorite chair. Loosen any restrictive clothing.
3. Start relaxing with several abdominal breaths; breathe in to the count of four, then breathe out to the count of eight.
4. Take a deep breath through your nose and hold it. Tense your feet as long as you can. (*Warning:* If you have a history of heart disease, high blood pressure, or stroke, consult your physician about this technique. He or she may suggest a modified version, with little or no breath-holding.)
5. Relax your feet as you exhale with a sigh through your mouth.
6. Take a few abdominal breaths, as in step 3.
7. Breathe in deeply through your nose. Hold it. Tense your calves.
8. Relax your calves as you breathe out with a strong exhalation.
9. Repeat the sequence for each area of the body, working from the extremities to the center: feet, calves, thighs, buttocks, abdomen. Next, the upper body: fingers, forearms, upper arms, shoulders. (Hunch your shoulders up to your ears.) Don't forget your face; it may hold much tension. Work it in three stages: pull your jaw back so your mouth looks funny, scrunch up your nose, furrow your brows.
10. Take a few minutes to relax and let go.[12]

I have found listening to tapes that take me through this relaxation exercise step by step very useful.

---

[12] Faelton, Sharon, and David Diamond, *Tension Turnaround* (Emmaus, Pa.: Rodale Press, 1990), p. 61.

This relaxation exercise can be very helpful in reducing tension and speeding up recovery. I recently worked with Judy, a twenty-eight-year-old mother and housewife. She had had neck pain for about five years, and upper back and left shoulder pain and numbness in her left arm for three months. She also experienced occasional lower back pain, knee pain, and pain in her feet and shins. She suffered intermittently from episodes of high blood pressure, for which she occasionally took medication. Judy was diagnosed with scoliosis as the cause of her back pain. Every morning her husband had to massage her back to relieve the pain.

When I explained to her my experiences and TMS, she understood perfectly well that her pain was caused by tension. However, she found it difficult to believe that positive self-talk and visualization could actually help her. Despite her skepticism, she applied the techniques and improved enough overnight not to require the morning massages from her husband.

Unfortunately, Judy was not motivated and did not take the recovery plan seriously. However, when she began to listen to a tape of the relaxation exercise described above and practiced it, she began to improve. She found this exercise quite helpful in relieving the pain.

Later I shared with her and her husband the strategies for good communication explained in Chapter Seven. As they began to communicate more, she was on her way to complete recovery. When I called her about four weeks later she had less pain and numbness; and eight weeks later she reported no more numbness in her arms and being almost completely pain-free. She said, "When the pain comes, I just keep telling it to go away and it does." Her blood pressure had become normal, and by all indications she was leading a healthier and happier life.

ACTION ITEM
Practice deep abdominal breathing and the relaxation exercise described above as much as possible. Get *The Five Keys to Permanent Stress Reduction* audio tapes and practice the relaxation methods mentioned on the tapes.[13]

As you see, these relaxation exercises are simple and easy to do. However, they can truly facilitate your recovery and your overall health and well-being. So make time in your daily schedule to take a few minutes and do them, especially in the first few days of your recovery.

4. Goal Setting

A famous study on goal setting, conducted at Yale University in 1953, is cited by almost every expert on this matter. This study discovered that only 3 percent of the graduating class that year had specific written goals and a plan for achieving them. In 1973, twenty years later, the same graduates were interviewed. The researchers discovered that those 3 percent were worth more financially than the other 97 percent combined. They were also found to enjoy a much higher level of happiness and joy in their lives. Setting and keeping goals is a powerful technique used by Olympic athletes as well as high achievers. Writing down our goals can make a tremendous difference in our success or failure in conquering pain.

To succeed in your fight against pain, you must make a list of things you yearn to accomplish in the next few hours, days, and weeks. As mentioned earlier, I began with short-term goals, such as walking in my home without shoes, and long-term goals of being able to carry my children without pain and taking karate lessons in two months. Fortunately, due to previous experiences

---

[13] Fiore, Neil and Lloyd Glauberman, *The Five Keys to Permanent Stress Reduction* (Los Angeles: Audio Renaissance Tapes, 1990), (800) 221-7945. In Chapter Seven you will find more information on how to relax.

with achieving my goals, I was able to do it, by the grace of God, in less than two weeks. Others who have set goals have experienced similar results.

You need to set goals in two categories: 1. short-term or daily goals; 2. long-term or ultimate goals.

Short-Term Goals. These goals are meant to help increase your mobility day by day and release you from the bondage of pain and disability in gradual, yet planned, steps.

ACTION ITEM

In your mind, make a list of positions and activities that are difficult for you due to pain. Include the amount of time you can stay in each position and the level of restriction on each activity. Then, set your short-term goals—that every day you will stay in those positions a few minutes longer and do more of those activities until complete recovery.

For example, let's assume you can only sit for fifteen minutes, stand five minutes, walk ten minutes, and climb two steps. Begin with the safest and easiest of these; set your goal to sit for eighteen to twenty minutes in the next twenty-four hours and to sit three to five minutes longer each day during the coming week. Once you have done this for a day or two and have become more confident in your ability to fight back pain, then you can set other short-term goals. The key is consistent improvement, no matter how small it may seem.

As demonstrated in my case and the experiences of others who have set such goals, it is quite possible to achieve your short-term goals easily and progress much more quickly than expected. However, do not try to do too much too soon; this may lead to more pain than you expected and delay your recovery.

Case in point: Harry, a friend of mine who is an mechanical engineer in his fifties, began having back pain while shoveling snow in Chicago eighteen years ago. He had received many different treatments with no success. Recently his condition had worsened. The pain was radiating into his legs, and his mid-back was also hurting. Harry had difficulty standing or walking for more than ten minutes and suffered the common restrictions that come with chronic back pain. He understood the concept of TMS, and as I explained the recovery plan to him he became quite excited. I helped him to design his own recovery plan, set goals, and choose ice cream as his reward.

The next day Harry walked thirty minutes instead of the fifteen minutes we had set as his short-term goal. He was able to stand and sit longer. He became quite excited about his small victory over eighteen years of back pain and celebrated with a taste of his favorite ice cream. However, since he had done so well, that night he decided to do his regular back exercises. These were the same ones he used to do for his back pain, and as this perhaps triggered memories of back pain on the subconscious level, he began to feel pain. The pain persisted and grew worse as Harry worried about it and criticized himself for pushing too hard. He had to spend part of the following day in bed. The story does have a happy ending. Since he was convinced that tension was responsible for the pain, he continued with the recovery plan, achieved his goal of jogging for about fifteen minutes in two weeks, and eventually recovered.

Keep in mind that as long as you are moving in the direction of becoming pain-free and increasing your level of activity, you are on the right track. Do not disappoint and overwhelm yourself by setting too many goals and not being able to achieve them. As I said earlier, for faster recovery, relax and enjoy yourself.

Now for those of you who are afraid of pushing against the pain, you have probably already done this many times. Consider the following point: It is quite common for people with chronic back pain to be in situations that require them to ignore and push back pain. It happens during a visit to the doctor or therapist, when you wait on uncomfortable seats. All the while, you have to endure extra pain. It could also happen at home or work, while taking care of children, doing your job, or on many other occasions.

However, now you are no longer just a helpless victim of

pain. You are in charge and are playing around with it—like a lion or a lioness playing around with a mouse. You already know that the inner child is resistant to change, and to maintain the pain habit and get your attention, it may increase the pain or move it to another part of your body, so do not let these developments alarm you.

Remember your symbol of power. Now close your eyes, take a deep breath, concentrate, and imagine yourself becoming your symbol of power. Strong and powerful. Now imagine your pain as something tiny over which you have full control. You can do whatever you want to it. YOU become BIGGER and STRONGER while your pain becomes smaller and weaker. Imagine this for a few moments and notice where in your body you feel strength and power. Now intensify those feelings in your mind and in wherever you feel them in your body. Do this at least five times.

Long-Term Goals. I like to call these your ultimate goals. They serve a double purpose. They keep you excited and motivated about your recovery as well as establish a high level of physical activity. If your ultimate goals include skiing, playing tennis, weight lifting, taking karate lessons, or taking a nice long vacation in Hawaii, you will be much more excited about your recovery. You can and should have several ultimate goals for the coming weeks and months; however, be sure that most of these goals help you achieve a higher level of physical activity.

ACTION ITEM

Now think of all those activities you yearn to do as your long-term goals and set a reasonable timetable for achieving them.

It is always more effective to be pulled toward a goal than pushed. If you know that by continuing with this challenge you could be skiing or playing tennis in thirty days, you will be much more eager to succeed.

At the end of this chapter you will find an easy-to-follow action plan with a progress chart in order to help you set goals, record your progress, and celebrate your accomplishments.

5. Reward and Punishment

As mentioned earlier, my experience has shown that the subconscious mind has the traits of a preschooler. From my perspective, Dr. Sarno's treatment relies on ignoring the misbehaving child and repeating certain phrases, such as "The pain is due to TMS, not to a structural abnormality," and "I must think psychological at all times, not physical. There is nothing wrong with my back." As with any child, he or she will stop misbehaving after being ignored long enough. Sometimes, to get your attention, he or she might hit you on the head or kick you in the knee and cause pain, but if you are patient enough, he or she will eventually give up.

However, how do you get a preschooler to cooperate with you and carry out your orders quickly? Give a reward! Setting a reward system can make the little child inside us all much more cooperative. It gives us something pleasurable to look forward to. This is such a simple way of focusing on something positive and enjoying at least a part of your day. I meet many people who find choosing a reward difficult and who have to think a long time to come up with an answer. If you find yourself in this category, now you know one of the reasons why tension builds up in you and causes pain. You need to take a few minutes a day and reward yourself.

Now what types of rewards should you choose? It is best to choose something that the little child in you really likes. Yummy treats like ice cream and cookies are a good start, but you need to look at what really excites the child in you. It could be a train ride, a hot bath, a new baseball cap, or a stuffed animal!

So you make a deal that if it doesn't cause you any pain, you will give the child its treat. I recommend you begin with some sort of sweet dessert item, such as ice cream, as a reward, since food treats tend to be more tied to our basic needs and stimulate our senses of smell, sight, and taste. Since we are dealing with negative emotions as causes of pain, strong positive emotions that are associated with our senses and basic needs are effective in eliminating the pain. Be creative and reward yourself by having your treat in a special setting, such as a quiet room, a nice restaurant, or in the park.

Think about your reward all day and imagine how wonderful it will taste, and see yourself enjoying and relishing every bite.[14]

I hope you will never have to punish your inner child, but it must be considered as a serious possibility. What do little children hate to do? Cleaning their rooms or other such chores. For me, cleaning the bathroom or my car's engine are real punishments.

Once you have punished your inner child in this way, it is amazing how the mere threat of punishment can make it listen to your orders and stop the pain. You can also use the threat of increasing the pain if your inner child gives you pain. As in my case and John's case, who was in a car accident, this strategy can be quite effective in getting your inner child to cooperate. I think the threat of inflicting pain on purpose triggers the pain-avoidance mechanism in the subconscious mind and overrules TMS.

However, as with most little children, a reward is usually better liked and more effective than punishment. Once you have

---

[14] As demonstrated from my own experience, this method can work very effectively to overcome back pain and hay fever. I have also used it to stop other TMS equivalents and negative thought patterns.

established a pattern, you can eliminate the need for a reward and simply give the order.

ACTION ITEM
Choose a reward that makes you excited about recovery.

Now say to the little child in you, "If you let me sit for thirty minutes without pain (or any other activity of your choice), I will give you _____." Then imagine achieving your desired result and enjoying your reward fully at least five times.

Certainly there are times when that little child cannot be persuaded by reward or punishment and he or she throws a temper tantrum. In such cases it might be necessary to simply ignore it for a while until it gives up.

6. Daily Record

Keep a daily record of your progress and accomplishments and review it every night. This provides you with daily feedback on your progress. It is also a very effective way to keep you focused and help dispel any doubts that might come to your mind during the initial stages of your recovery. As mentioned earlier, I experienced just such doubts in the first few days of my recovery; however, a quick review of my accomplishments helped me stay confident in the diagnosis and the recovery program and dispelled any doubts.

The above six steps are essential for rapid recovery. The following three steps will help you continue on your path to a pain-free and active life.

7. Exercise

Exercise is vital to everyone's general health and well-being. It is extremely important in continuing your progress toward a pain-free body. Besides releasing tension and helping you relax, regular exercise gives you a sense of well-being and helps build confidence in your physical abilities. It also provides you with more strength and stamina.

In addition to regular aerobic exercise, such as walking or swimming, working out with weights is an excellent way to build your confidence. Many back-pain sufferers are led to believe that their pain is due to weak muscles and are told that lifting or carrying heavy objects is bad for the back. Also, after many months and years of bed rest and restricted activity, you might feel physically weak and incapable of lifting or carrying heavy objects. To overcome this, the best approach is to challenge this false notion of weakness with a weight training program.

You may consult a certified athletic trainer, a book, or a video on weight training to make sure you are using correct form when working out.[15] I started with very light weights and soon felt so strong and confident that I carried both my children, each weighing more than forty pounds.

NOTE: Many people think of bodybuilders when weight training is mentioned. However, studies have shown that regular weight training helps in maintaining and improving health and disease prevention. In a number of studies, senior citizens in their eighties and nineties were able to increase their strength by 200-300 percent and live more independently after just a few weeks of weight training.[16]

Also, some people tend to make weight training a challenge. But remember, weight training should be done for confidence building and fun while you are recovering. If you find yourself too anxious to move to higher weights and it is becoming frustrating,

---

[15] Bill Pearl, *Getting Stronger: Weight Training for Men and Women* (Bolinas, Calif.: Shelter Publishing Company, 1986) is among the many books you will find in your local library or bookstore that provide a good, safe, basic workout program. Consult your physician if you suffer from heart disease or other disorders that would require proper modifications for a safe exercise program.

[16] For more detail see *Biomarkers: The 10 Keys to Prolonging Vitality*, by Dr. William J. Evans (New York: Fireside Books, 1991).

it will become a new source of stress. Believe me, I am talking from experience. You are not preparing for the Olympics, so take it easy and do it for the fun of it.

CAUTION: Keep in mind that performing back exercises as a treatment measure or for preventing back pain means that you are focusing on the problem and can lead to persistence or recurrence of pain. You must exercise for enjoyment and to build your confidence. This is a wonderful way to relax and remain pain-free.

8. Self-Discipline

It is very important to have self-discipline to remain pain-free. With self-control and self-discipline you can guide all your resources toward accomplishing your goals. One of the best ways to develop self-discipline is to set certain daily tasks that have to be done regardless of how busy you are or tired you feel. Accomplishing these tasks proves to yourself and to your mind that when you take up a task, you will do it and continue doing it day after day, no matter what obstacles you have to face. These simple tasks help strengthen your willpower and make it easier to succeed in reaching your goals.

ACTION ITEM
Consider a number of simple daily tasks you must do for developing a higher level of self-discipline.

These can be simple tasks, from taking ten deep breaths and brushing your teeth to the count of 100, to dusting the table and making your bed. You be the judge of what assignments to give yourself, based on your level of pain and ability to move. As these tasks become easier, you can make them more challenging and do them under more difficult conditions, such as doing them at an exact time of day or in a better way.

9. Desensitization and Positive Association

These are the processes that enable a person to interact with an object or a situation that brings about a great deal of fear and anxiety.

Someone who has been in a horrible car accident may find it very difficult to even hear the word car, much less to drive one. Using the desensitization process, the person is gradually reintroduced to the car under favorable circumstances. When he or she is relaxed, the word car is mentioned in a story about a wonderful vacation, or a picture of a car is shown to the person. Later, he or she is asked to look at a car from the comfort and security of home, and eventually to sit and be driven in one. Based on the person's progress and tolerance of each step, in a matter of days or weeks he or she might once again be able to drive a car without feeling afraid or anxious.

In this example, the person was first reintroduced to the car in a relaxed, comfortable environment through a story about an enjoyable vacation. This is called positive association—that is, associating what has become a negative experience with a positive one until it no longer causes fear or anxiety.

Exactly the same principle can be applied to back-related terminology. If words such as disc, pain, or sciatica trigger a negative response both emotionally and physically by causing pain when they are mentioned, this method can help. Using the desensitization process in a relaxed, comfortable state, think of or say the word that is least painful. Later that day, or on the next day, repeat that word two or three times. Eventually it loses its pain-causing effect.

Sometimes hearing a word is more painful than saying it. In that case, you can tape the word and listen to it. However, most people do not use these words in their daily lives. So unless these words are related to your daily routine, you may not need to use these methods.

PUTTING IT ALL TOGETHER

Now it is time to incorporate the nine steps into an easy-to-follow recovery plan. As you have seen, these techniques are easy, fun, quite effective, and take little time to do. For example, the positive thinking strategy requires that you to take a minute and tell yourself before sleep that you are not going to hurt any more and visualize yourself as being healthy and strong. However, if you have never done this, like anything new, it may require some effort on your part to remember to do it. That is why it is extremely crucial for you to take a few minutes and design your recovery plan. It may take you twenty minutes or so to follow the steps in this section and design a daily action plan, but this is a very small price to pay for recovery. Compare this to how much time it takes to make an appointment to see the doctor, chiropractor, or therapist, drive to his or her office, wait there to be examined or treated, and drive home over and over again.

The following program is designed for a patient with chronic back or neck pain who is severely restricted in his or her daily activities. You may make appropriate changes to suit your particular condition. I recommend that you read the entire action plan first so that you have an overview of what you need to do and then follow it step by step. **Remember to apply these strategies with the belief and intention that they will help you to recover completely and rapidly.**

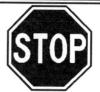

Now I want you to take a moment and again make the intention for rapid recovery. I want you to close your eyes, focus your mind, and make the intention in your heart and in your mind that every action you take now will help you recover rapidly. You might want to say to yourself,

"Every step I take from now on will help me to recover faster and faster."

Make a fist and say it with a serious expression on your face. Say it to yourself several times with feeling and determination. No matter what happens, you are determined to overcome your pain and live pain-free.[17]

DESIGNING YOUR RECOVERY PLAN

Preparation

Location and Time. Choose a place and a time that will give you about twenty minutes to yourself. No phone calls, kids, or interruptions. This will allow you to concentrate on designing your recovery plan.

Motivation. If you have read this far, I assume you are quite

---

[17] I oftentimes ask people to think of their recovery as a trip to a wonderful vacation destination. On the way they may experience problems, such as a flat tire, but such problems do not cause them to give up their plans and return home. They simply change the tire and continue on vacation. On your way to recovery you may also experience certain difficulties, but as long as you have made up your mind to become pain-free and healthy and do not give up, you can expect to reach your goal.

motivated to recover. If you feel you need to become more motivated, however, write down a list of events and opportunities you have missed in the past, are missing now, and will miss in the future due to chronic back or neck pain, in any of the following categories: personal, social, professional, financial, educational, or any other category you feel necessary. Use the following chart to write down one missed opportunity in each category.

NOTE: If you find this process too painful to do and/or feel you are already motivated enough to begin your recovery immediately move on to the benefits and pleasures of rapid recovery.

OPPORTUNITIES LOST DUE TO CHRONIC PAIN			
	Past	Present	Future
Personal	*my wife*	*my wife*	*my wife*
Social	*Bikdg*	*Biking*	*Bik.*
Professional	*No Work*	*no work*	*No Work*
Financial			
Educational			

I know that writing down these missed opportunities, whether it was your child's school play, a promotion at work, or attending a friend's wedding, can be quite painful. However, by increasing the level of pain you attach to this condition, you put yourself in a much stronger position for recovery than before. Unfortunately, I have met people who have become "accustomed" to living with pain and the restrictions it brings as a normal part of their lives. This exercise helps to put pain and disability in its proper perspective.

Take a hard look at this list, close your eyes, and remember how sad you felt. Then get mad and make up your mind that you are sick and tired of being in pain, and you are not going to take it any more. Do it now!

In order to increase your level of motivation for rapid recovery, you also need to attach as much pleasure as possible to living healthy and pain-free. In the chart below write down all the benefits and pleasures you associate with rapid recovery

BENEFITS AND PLEASURES OF RECOVERING FROM PAIN	
Personal	
Social	
Professional	
Financial	
Educational	

These tables are reproduced in Appendix A. You can transfer your information into those tables, cut them out, and post them by your bed or mirror. They will be a constant reminder during your recovery that you can no longer afford to live with pain and disability. DO IT NOW!

Goals. Now you need to make a list of short-term daily goals designed to increase your level of activity in gradual and careful steps. These goals will help you get back to your normal activity level in a few days.

Begin by writing down in the progress chart on the next page how much longer you would like to stay in a particular position for the next twenty-four hours and during the following six days after that. Since most people who have followed the nine-step recovery plan have been able to achieve their goals faster than expected, I recommend using a pencil to write down your goals. This way you can change them to fit your speed of recovery.

Choose an easy to achieve number, such as five or ten minutes longer. If you are very restricted note how long you can sit or stand and increase the time a little beyond the point you are able to tolerate the pain. Then add that many minutes to the following days so that by the end of one week you can sit or stand an extra thirty to sixty minutes. For bending, choose the number of degrees you want to be able to bend for the first twenty-four hours and add a few more degrees to it for the following six days. If you choose ten degrees and you cannot bend at all right now, you should be able to bend almost ninety degrees by the end of the week.

If you are experiencing chronic pain and restricted movement in your shoulder and neck, or arms and hands, you may set goals to improve in those areas.

You may use the blank rows to set additional goals. Do not be surprised to see that you have easily surpassed your goals. Many people have.

SHORT-TERM GOALS							
	1	2	3	4	5	6	7
GOAL							
Sit							
Stand							
Bend							

Now it's time to set your reward. Choose a reward that is easy to acquire and gives you a lot of pleasure. When you are done choosing your reward, write it down in the space below.

My Reward

Make sure to reward yourself as soon as your goals are achieved. If you want rapid recovery, do not postpone it. As a part of preparation for your recovery get your reward and have it readily available (ice cream waiting in the freezer, for example). Its mental and emotional impact is greater than you think.

You are provided with a progress chart in Appendix A. Transfer your goal and reward information there, cut it out, and post it next to your bed or on a mirror so that you can see it every night and every morning. Think about your goals and your reward all day. The more you focus on them, the sooner you can achieve them.

Now take a moment, close your eyes, take a deep breath, hold it for a moment, and exhale with a sigh of relief—aaaaahhhh. Now visualize yourself sitting, standing, and bending easily and comfortably, and feeling great. See yourself getting your reward and enjoying it fully.

To become more motivated, visualize how being able to achieve your short-term goals will assist you to engage in some of the activities that you yearn to do, but have not been able to accomplish due to chronic pain. Think of a time in the next two to four weeks when you want to be able to participate in those activities, whether it's carrying your children, playing tennis, or taking a vacation. You will have an opportunity to write them down in your ultimate goals chart shortly.

If you have access to a library or a bookstore, try to get books, audiotapes, or videotapes on mind/body medicine and healing. I strongly recommend that you read Dr. Sarno's *Mind over Back Pain* and *Healing Back Pain* if you have not done so. *Anatomy of an Illness* and *Head First: The Biology of Hope* by Norman Cousins and *Healing and the Mind by Bill Moyers*[18] are also appropriate reading for this stage of recovery, as they give you a better understanding of the immense potential we all have to utilize our innate abilities to recover from serious and chronic disorders. Always tell yourself: If others in much worse condition have been able to recover, so can I.

IMPLEMENTATION

Now that you have clear goals, it is time for positive thinking and mental exercises. At night before sleep, while lying in bed, take a deep breath, hold it for a few moments, concentrate, then exhale and say to yourself, "I am not going to hurt any more. I will certainly win my battle against pain. No TMS or subconscious mind is going to stop me from living a healthy, active life now."

---

[18] Videotapes of *Healing and the Mind* might be available at your local library or bookstore. If not, you can order them through Public Television Station WNET, (800) 336-1917, or by calling Ambrose Video Production, (800) 526-4663.

If you like to use a different phrase, write it down in the space below.

_____

Say this at least five times and do it with a positive, determined attitude, a serious expression on your face, and clenched fists. Set your mind and your intention that all the steps you are taking will lead to your complete recovery.

Now use the space below to write down your symbol of power and strength.

_____

Visualize yourself becoming your symbol of power winning a competition or a battle. Relive a time or an activity when you felt strong, powerful, and unstoppable. If you cannot think of one, imagine the kind of activity or situation that would make you feel strong and powerful.

See the subconscious mind as an opponent with whom you have been wrestling for months and losing every time. But this time you are going to defeat it and win back your health. You throw it on the ground, hear it hitting it hard, so hard that the ground shakes. Do it several times, and each time feel stronger than before. Try to see this scene in as much detail as possible and in color. Hear the sounds you associate with victory and triumph. Be the hero of your own mental movie.[19]

After you have defeated your pain opponent, see yourself achieving your goals easily and quickly. See yourself sitting or standing for hours doing your favorite activities, and bending and touching the floor without feeling any pain or discomfort. In fact, go on a mental vacation where you are bending and picking flowers from a garden and giving them to your loved ones, sitting on the beach and watching the sunset, and standing on the peak

---

[19] If you need more clarification on any of these strategies, you may refer to the section on the strategy in question.

of a mountain, breathing in cool fresh air and looking at the beautiful valley below. See the sights, hear the sounds, and feel the feelings. Do this enough times to see things in color and in great detail.[20]

RECOVERY BEGINS

Day One

As with most people who have applied these strategies, chances are this morning you woke up with less pain and discomfort. You slept better than previous nights and are excited and ready to take back your life.

Before you get out of bed, visualize yourself as strong and powerful, like a sleeping giant waking up from a long sleep. Imagine your feet and hands are gigantic; every step you take shakes the ground and your steps can be heard from miles away. The sound of your steps and the ground shaking wakes up the entire town, and people are calling the radio and TV stations to report this unusual event. The tiny subconscious has no chance of standing in your way to a healthy, active life now.

Now you are ready to get out of bed and face the day. You are feeling energized and much more confident about your ability to beat the pain. Greet yourself with an enthusiastic good morning and think about how wonderful getting your reward will feel. Tell your little subconscious that the only way he or she will get the reward is by cooperating with you to achieve your goals easily and quickly. Take a few moments and visualize yourself

---

[20] If you do not want to wait till night time to begin positive self-talk and visualization, you can start doing them right away. It works best if you can do them when there are no interruptions and you can focus all your thoughts on them. One way to do this is by lying down or sitting comfortably in a quiet place, taking several deep breaths, then doing them. However, before sleep is an optimum time to communicate to your subconscious, so be sure to talk to your mind and visualize at that time as well.

achieving your goals easily and with great results.

Remember to put your body into it. Your posture is very important. As much as you can during the day, **practice positive thinking, sit erect, and stand tall. Act strong and tough by putting more energy into whatever you do. See yourself become a lion or a lioness, a steam engine, or whatever your symbol of power is. Show your subconscious mind that you are in charge now. This is body over mind.**

When the time comes to achieve your goal, approach it with a calm and confident attitude. Like a parent who knows exactly how to deal with a misbehaving child, remember that action speaks louder than words. As you sit or stand for those extra few minutes, do not back down when the pain begins. Instead of becoming worried and thinking negatively, focus on your reward and the images of power and strength that you have been visualizing. See yourself as a large tree, with your roots going hundreds of feet into the ground. You are firmly established in your place, and no pain is going to make you get up. Be confident that like thousands of people who have recovered from chronic back pain, you can beat the pain, too. Do not shift around. Stay in one position like that large tree!

Now remember the focusing exercise you did earlier, where you chose a word to focus your mind on. This is a good time to do it. This helps you to take conscious control of your thoughts and concentrate your energy on recovery. Focus your eyes on a particular object for a few seconds while thinking of a word that you associate with positive feelings. By focusing your eyes and mind on a particular object and thought, you are disciplining your subconscious mind to be obedient to your conscious desires and commands.

NOTE: Do not be surprised if the pain moves to another part of your body or intensifies temporarily. Also, it is possible to experience other physical manifestations of tension, such as stomach problems, eczema, hay fever, headache, etc., as the subconscious tries to attract your attention to some other physical problem. You might want to read Chapter Seven: "The Road to

Wellness" now. By knowing how to communicate properly and learning about the stress-coping strategies, you will feel empowered and experience less of these symptoms.

After you achieve your goals for the first day, congratulate yourself. Give yourself a pat on the back and give your inner child the reward it has been waiting for. Make this a very special occasion. Do it in a setting where there are no interruptions and you can enjoy every moment. Take your time. *As mentioned earlier, do not postpone this step if you yearn for rapid recovery.*

Make sure to record your actual achievement on the progress chart. "Congratulations! You have made it through the first day. Thank you for your cooperation. I knew you could do it." This is what you will say to your subconscious as you record your achievements.

If you have progressed like most people I have worked with, you are ready to expand your short-term goals now. Use the chart on the next page to set new goals related to your daily activities. In addition to the activities listed, you can add any activity appropriate for your particular condition in the space provided.

Based on how long you can walk, how many steps you can climb, and how many pounds you can carry, set your goals for the next day to push these limits and do a little more of each.

Choose a reward as before. When you are done choosing your reward, write it down in the space below.

My Reward

Remember to transfer this information to the chart in Appendix A and post it as before.

At night before sleep review your accomplishments, congratulate yourself for even the smallest improvement, and visualize achieving your goals for the next day with complete ease, then really enjoying your reward.

ADVANCED SHORT-TERM GOALS						
1	2	3	4	5	6	7
GOAL						
Walk						
Climb						
Carry						

Practice the progressive relaxation technique mentioned in the strategy on mental exercises. This involves taking deep breaths and tightening various muscle groups, holding the breath and the tension in those muscles, and then exhaling and relaxing the muscles at the same time. This is an excellent way to release any unnoticed tension in your muscles before sleep. Whenever I do this I get a very deep, restful sleep.

By the way, one important point to consider: The mind needs time to adjust to these improvements in your health. Overnight improvement of a chronic, painful, and debilitating condition may be difficult for your mind to accept. In other words, as you begin to sit longer, bend more, and do the other things you were not able to do less than twenty-four hours earlier (and for so many weeks or months), your mind may have some difficulty adjusting to these new changes. Since you already know that many others have rapidly recovered, do not be overwhelmed by your accomplishments, just continue with your recovery plan. As you improve step by step each day, very soon your mind will come to accept this new level of activity on your part. Again, this is where visualization plays a crucial part to help your mind and body work in harmony toward achieving your goals.

Day Two

Good morning! If you have progressed as planned, you are feeling a new sense of life and energy. Everything looks new and beautiful. You are feeling alive again.[21]

This morning you may give some positive reinforcement to your subconscious mind by staying under the shower a little longer, having something special for breakfast, or enjoying a tasty snack between meals. When you do any of these, tell your inner child that the only reason you do this is because he or she has been cooperating with you, and more goodies are on the way if you recover as planned.

Continue your march toward recovery by giving yourself the proper images of health and power and body postures that clearly show you are confident and unstoppable. Keep thinking about your reward and how wonderful it will taste or feel. Again visualize achieving your goals, and practice focusing on them. Be confident of your ability to achieve them and overcome your disability.

Next comes achieving your advanced short-term goals. Again, approach this effort with a calm and confident attitude. Do the easier activities first, such as walking a few minutes or a few steps longer. As you build your confidence in your physical abilities, try meeting your other goals. Do not do too much too soon. It is very exciting to improve so quickly after months or years of disability, and you might want to do it all. However, you have been conditioned to feel pain and, like a bad habit, the conditioning needs to be broken in gradual and planned steps.

The mechanical engineer mentioned earlier was able to walk for thirty minutes on his first day of recovery; that was twice his

---

[21] If you have not improved as planned, continue with your goals for the first day. Be persistent and don't give up easily. You might want to try setting a punishment for your inner child if it does not cooperate, or try to scare the pain away as I explained earlier. Use strong positive emotions to fight back negative emotions.

goal and three times what he could do one day earlier. However, he got too excited, did a lot of stretches and exercises that night, and caused himself too much pain. This delayed his recovery by a day or two. So follow your recovery as planned; if you were able to walk more or climb more than expected, be happy and celebrate your progress. Whether you are functioning at full capacity in three days or eight, you have recovered faster than most conventional treatments for chronic back pain would permit.

In addition to achieving your advanced short-term goals, continue to sit and stand longer and do more of your previous short-term goals. You might try sitting on different chairs or on the sofa. Stand with slippers on instead of shoes. Try doing things by relaxing some of the restrictions placed on you by pain and conditioning. Always use good judgment.

After you achieve your goals, congratulate yourself, even pat yourself on the back, and reward yourself. Be creative in the way you reward yourself. If the reward is ice cream, maybe add a topping to it, or go somewhere special and eat it. Take your time when doing it and keep telling your inner child how proud you are of your work together as a team.

Record your actual achievement on the progress chart. Continue with positive self-talk. If you have recovered better than planned, give an extra reward to your inner child as positive reinforcement. This could be anything from taking a long hot bath to playing a game.

Now it is time to set some ultimate goals for yourself, goals that propel you toward complete recovery and put you as far away as possible from what your physical condition was before. These goals make you excited and keep you motivated to continue on your recovery plan.

First make a list of activities you yearn to do in the next few weeks. Write them down without considering your present abilities, or should I say disabilities. They could be participating in sports such as tennis, golf, weight lifting, or swimming. They could relate to your children playing with them, carrying them, or taking them to an amusement park. They could be eating at your favorite restaurant, taking a well-deserved vacation, or visiting friends. Whatever you decide to do, write them all down on a sheet of paper and then, based on your progress so far, evaluate when you will be most likely to achieve your ultimate goals. Place a 1 in front of those things you wish to do by the end of the first week of your recovery, which is five days from now, and 2, 3, or 4 for others you want to do.

Now in the chart on the next page write down your ultimate goal or goals. If some of your goals need more than four weeks you have space for those as well. Just remember to choose goals that are very likely for you to achieve. Aim high, but set reasonable, achievable goals.[22]

Again remember to transfer the above information to the chart in Appendix A and post it.

You might want to set a reward for achieving these goals as well, but these are activities that you yearn to do anyway. Just being able to engage in them is very rewarding in itself.

Again at night, before sleep, review your accomplishments for the day and ever since you began your recovery. Congratulate yourself and feel good all over. Visualize improving in reducing your level of pain, increasing your physical activities, and meeting your short-term goals. Also, visualize achieving your ultimate goals and how fantastic you will feel when you do.

---

[22] Once I was showing a forty-two-year-old electrical engineer, who had recovered overnight from chronic pain in his chest using my nine-step recovery plan, how to work out with light weights. I told him that once these weights were too easy for him, he could get heavier ones and eventually use a barbell. He smiled and said, "Barbell! I don't think I'll ever get to that level in weight training."

"Set your goals high so that you can reach your full potential," I told him. See every achievement as a stepping stone to bigger ones. Strike a balance between being happy and content with what you have achieved so far, no matter how big or small, and looking forward to accomplishing even more soon. Do not aim so low that you do not reach your full potential, or aim so high that you criticize yourself for not achieving your goals. Aim just beyond your reach, so that you can stretch and strengthen your abilities.

ULTIMATE LONG-TERM GOALS			
	GOAL ONE	GOAL TWO	GOAL THREE	GOAL FOUR
WEEK			
One			
Two			
Three			
Four			

Day Three

At this point you need to evaluate your progress and reevaluate your goals. If you have improved as fast as most people who have followed my nine-step recovery plan, you are ready to increase your short-term goals in time or set new ones. If you have not improved as expected, do not give up. Know that persistence pays off.

Today, besides positive thinking, mental exercises, and meeting your goals, plan on increasing your level of activity. You might want to add one or two daily tasks to what you are already doing for self-discipline, such as taking ten deep breaths or brushing your teeth to the count of one hundred. These tasks should be done regardless of how busy you are or how tired you feel. In this way you show your inner child that you are serious about your recovery, and that when you decide to do something consistently and in a persistent manner, you will definitely do it.

Days Four–Six

During this period, continue with your recovery as planned but also try to start a light exercise program. You can begin with simply going for a short walk or a swim. As you feel more comfortable with your exercise routine and confident about your physical abilities, introduce weight training into your routine. Weight training does a lot to boost your confidence in your physical abilities. You may consult an athletic trainer or a book on weight training. Begin a strengthening routine for your arms, chest, shoulders, and leg muscles. Feel free to add pushups and sit-ups to your routine as well. Do not be in a rush to move on to heavier weights. The purpose here is to build your self-confidence, not prepare you for the state weight-lifting championships. Take your time and you will see the physical and mental benefits of exercise soon enough.

Day Seven

Now we have come to the end of your first week of recovery. I strongly recommend that you reward yourself in a special way for your accomplishments so far. How about a new set of clothes, dinner at a fine restaurant, or a hot bath? I hope the one thing you have realized since beginning your recovery is the need to take better care of yourself. Whether it is having a few minutes to yourself to enjoy an ice cream or going for a short walk, it is important to give your mind and your body a chance to relax and enjoy life on a daily basis.

Most people I have worked with realize that if they do not set limits to how much they can take physically and/or emotionally, they could end up with chronic pain again. However, there were those who told me they did not have time to take a few minutes to exercise or relax. I reminded them of the many hours they had spent in bed with back pain or seeking treatment. It is simply a matter of prevention versus cure. So as you progress and begin to get back into life, keep in mind that even though you might not be able to change your circumstances, you can live a healthier life by taking better care of yourself.

In addition to rewarding yourself for your accomplishments for the week, you could also celebrate by achieving your ultimate goals for the end of the first week. Was it jogging ten minutes, or a weekend getaway? Whatever you had decided to do, I hope you will be successful in doing it and enjoy it immensely.

Days Eight–Fourteen

I believe by now you have practiced the steps and have progressed enough to be able to continue on your own. Remember to reevaluate your short-term and long-term goals based on your progress. If certain words related to your chronic pain trigger pain, you might want to read Step 9: Desensitization. It is a simple process, but it will help reduce the negative effects of those words on you.

By the end of this week you are ready to achieve your ultimate goals for the second week of your recovery and should be on your way to better health and a more enjoyable life.[23]

At this point I would like to share with you a few important points to help you attain complete recovery:

1. Keep in mind the importance of conditioning. Experts on behavior modification and habit formation say for an action to become firmly established in our minds we must practice it for three to four weeks. Thus, I highly recommend continuing with positive thinking, visualization, relaxation, and the other techniques. This is the best way to help you dispel any doubts and continue with your recovery. Do this for the next thirty days in order to firmly establish this new habit pattern of a pain-free body.

2. Take the time to keep a daily record, review your achievements, and keep yourself motivated to reach your goals, and stay confident.

3. I highly recommend that you become proactive and watch

---

[23] As demonstrated earlier, these steps were quite effective in eliminating my back pain and other tension-related symptoms. If you have used these methods before to reach your goals, you will find it easier to apply them to chronic back pain and accelerate your recovery. However, as with any recovery program, individual results may vary.

for times of stress and tension in your life. If your car broke down in the morning, you had an argument with your spouse, your kids are sick, and you are anxious about meeting an important deadline at work, talk to your subconscious at night before going to sleep. Say, "I have enough problems to deal with already; I do not want any trouble from you. Do you understand?" Then do as I do: I imagine sending him with his head down in defeat to his room and locking the door. This simple step helps reduce future episodes of back or neck pain. It has worked well for me.

4. Be aware of the fact that we live with stress and tension daily and that, as a result, you may experience some back or neck pain, especially as your condition improves and you return to full-time work and resume more family responsibilities. Do not be surprised by the pain, but see it as a signal that you may need to make some changes in the way you communicate your feelings to others or in your ways of handling anger, anxiety, stress, and tension.

These basic methods can help to subdue your little child subconscious in order to accelerate your recovery. They certainly worked for me and for others who have applied them. I hope they will work for you to help you recover rapidly from chronic back pain and eventually reach a point where you can stop TMS simply by commanding your subconscious to stop the pain.[24]

In the next chapter I will explain in detail the strategies and techniques that help me reduce or eliminate tension and, therefore, the cause of back pain.

---

[24] For more detailed explanation of the above methods the reader may consult *Introduction to Psychology,* by Rita Atkinson, et al. (New York: Harcourt Brace Jovanovich Publishers, 1990).

7

THE ROAD TO WELLNESS

*A*uthor Michael Crichton, in his autobiography *Travels,* wrote that prior to his decision to become a novelist he trained as a doctor at Harvard Medical School. During the time he spent on the cardiology ward, he asked the patients, "Why did you have a heart attack?" Here are some of the answers he was given:

"You really want to know. . . . I got a promotion. The company wants me to move to Cincinnati. But my wife doesn't want to go. She has all her family in Boston, and she doesn't want to go with me. That's why."

"My wife is talking about leaving me. . . ."

"My son won't go to law school."

"I want to get a divorce and I feel guilty."

"My wife wants another baby and I don't think we can afford it. . . ."

These patients were telling me stories of events that had affected their hearts in a metaphorical sense. They were telling me love stories. Sad love stories, which had pained their hearts. Their wives and families and bosses didn't care for them. Their hearts were attacked.

And pretty soon, their hearts were *literally* attacked. And they experienced physical pain. And that pain, that attack, was going to force a change in their lives, and the lives of those around them. . . . It made almost too much sense.[1]

Crichton's observation underscores what we intuitively know: Our relationship with our loved ones can have a grave effect on our emotional and physical health.

So far the focus of this book has been on pain and how to eliminate it. However, most back and neck pain are caused by tension, and unless we resolve the issues that lead to it, we are vulnerable to physical manifestations of tension in one form or another.[2]

As I helped others to recover from chronic back pain, most had no difficulty identifying the people and the circumstances that were sources of chronic tension in their lives. The problem was that they did not know how to deal with these situations in an effective and constructive manner and, as a result suffered a great deal of anger, anxiety, and frustration.

So in addition to explaining TMS and the nine-step recovery plan, I began to share with them the concepts and strategies that helped me to reduce and/or eliminate tension in various areas of my life. Hence, this chapter.

However, first I want to tell you about an empowering concept that I learned long ago through studying the lives of scientists and other important historical figures: There are no problems, only challenges and opportunities. This concept has helped me face many difficult situations by allowing me to see problems as challenges and opportunities to learn and grow.

---

[1] Michael Crichton, *Travels* (New York: Ballantine Books, 1988), pp. 62–63.

[2] I consider TMS and its equivalents early warning signs. If we do not pay attention to them and resolve the underlying issues that cause chronic anger, anxiety, frustration, and tension in our lives, we could suffer from more serious conditions, such as heart attacks, strokes, or cancer.

In addition to learning to become a more informed consumer and to utilize my mind's abilities for better health, one of the most important lessons I learned from tension-caused pain and disability was that I needed to make substantial changes in the way I handled my close relationships and those situations that were constant sources of anger and tension. Resolving those issues was the best way to eliminate tension, stress, and pain.

Here too I tried to benefit from the lessons I learned. I searched for new techniques and strategies for dealing with stressful relationships and situations and combined them with my knowledge of psychology and common sense to create a more harmonious and peaceful life. These strategies have helped me discharge my responsibilities and obligations as a husband and father in a better and more efficient way, by building consensus and teamwork within my family. Now many of the issues and tasks that used to be a great source of worry, concern, and tension are resolved and accomplished without overburdening myself beyond my limits, as used to be the case. As a constant perfectionist, I have to say that is quite a relief.

GOOD COMMUNICATION HELPS

When I learned how unconscious repression of my anger and anxiety had led to so much physical pain, I realized the enormous amount of negative feelings I was holding in and how ineffective I had been in communicating my feelings and expectations to my wife, parents, and others close to me. Although I had studied psychology, taken courses and workshops in communication, and have a job that requires communicating with hundreds of people, I was unaware of some very important aspects of effective communication. Since I learned them, I have found in my own life that good communication is one of the most important means to great relationships and a more peaceful, happier, and healthier life.

How to Do It

There are many books written about proper ways to communicate and open yourself to others, without getting hurt or hurting others' feelings, and how to establish rapport and good communication. Interestingly enough, I found the steps to good communication in books on health. In fact, good communication is so vital to our health and well being that Dr. Dean Ornish has made it an essential part of his scientifically proven program for reversing heart disease and has dedicated an entire chapter, "Opening Your Heart to Others," in his book on heart disease. I have found the following steps very helpful and effective in creating proper communication: [3]

1. Always choose an appropriate time.
2. Make it clear that you want to discuss something important.
3. Defuse the situation.
4. Identify what you are feeling.
5. Express your feelings.
6. Be specific, positive, and do not talk too much.
7. Never make assumptions; ask questions.
8. Be a concerned, compassionate listener.
9. Acknowledge what the other person is saying.

These steps appear quite simple and are common sense; however, oftentimes they are neglected. When we are angry and upset over an issue, we are very likely to disregard these steps and end up with more problems due to miscommunication. Other times we do not follow them because we have become conditioned to communicate with someone in a way that ignores these steps. And how about times when we take others for granted because they are our spouse, children, or subordinates, and expect them to pay full attention to everything we say and understand it the way we believe they should? These are some common reasons why proper communication steps are not followed, resulting in miscommunication, misunderstandings, and difficulties in relationships, whether at work or at home.

---

[3] These steps were adapted from *Dr. Dean Ornish's Program for Reversing Heart Disease* (Random House, 1991), pp. 203–208, and *Prevention Magazine's 30-Day Immune Power Program* (Rodale Books, 1992), pp. 204–205.

1. Always choose an appropriate time. Trying to discuss sensitive issues while the other person is busy is a sure way to create communication difficulties, whether it's your spouse who is busy cooking or your supervisor who is preparing for a meeting. What about talking to kids, or even adults, about something important while they are watching TV? Are they going to hear and understand much of what you say?

So choose a time and a place where there are no interruptions and you can share your concerns without distractions. If necessary, take time off from work, get a babysitter, or take any other needed steps in order to arrange an appropriate time to meet.

Meet when the other person is in a positive emotional state. If he or she just got a stressful phone call, that is definitely not the right time. Use good judgment and common sense in choosing the time.

2. Make it clear that you want to discuss something important. Let the other person know from the very beginning that what you have to say is very important to you and that you appreciate his or her patience in listening to you. If you do not make this clear, you may find the other person inattentive or in a hurry to leave for more important matters.

3. Defuse the situation. If the issue you want to discuss has been a sore point in the past, make it clear from the start that this is an important and sensitive matter that has caused or might cause anger or lead to an argument, but that you would really appreciate the other person's cooperation in listening to you. You must also promise to listen to his or her side when you are done explaining yours. This calm and open attitude helps, in most cases, to set up a favorable atmosphere for good communication.

I recommend choosing an issue that is not so sensitive as to provoke anger and hostility when you first begin to apply these strategies. Your first priority is to get into the habit of communicating properly with the other person, not to resolve all the issues that are sources of anger and frustration in one sitting!

After you have established good communication and the other person knows that you can talk about problems, and in most cases come up with a solution that is agreed to by both of you, your chances of resolving more sensitive issues are certainly much better. Use good judgment and common sense regarding which areas of the relationship you need to communicate about first.

4. Identify what you are feeling. This is extremely important and probably one of the major obstacles to good communication. In today's society most us are always in such a hurry to move on to the next task that we have lost touch with our feelings, not only on the psychological level but on the physical level as well.

We touch hundreds of objects daily, from pen and paper to our clothes and people's hands, yet we would have difficulty remembering and identifying how they feel. What is their texture, temperature, or make. The same is true of the food we eat. We are in such a hurry to finish our meals and our minds are so busy with worries, thoughts, or a TV show, that we do not really notice texture and taste of what we eat.[4]

On the psychological level this problem is even worse. We learn early on that not only showing but also *feeling* our feelings and emotions is a sign of weakness. Certainly there is a time and a place for showing our feelings and a time and a place when we should keep our feelings to ourselves. However, most of us have learned to repress our feelings to such an extent that we find it difficult to identify, much less to express, them.

Identifying our feelings is a very important aspect of good communication because sometimes it is difficult to distinguish between feelings, thoughts, and judgments. Feelings are true statements and represent the present. We may feel a certain way due to our upbringing and other reasons, and this is more easily understood and accepted by the other person than a thought or a judgment. When I say, "I am frustrated," or "I feel sad," no judgment or criticism of the other person is involved; it is simply a statement of

---

[4] When we learn to take a few moments to focus on what we are doing and pay attention to how we breathe, to feel the texture of our clothes, or to eat our food slowly, for a few minutes we free our minds from thoughts about the past and worries about the future. This is called mindfulness and is quite effective in helping us cope with the stresses of daily life.

fact. But this lets the other person know how their behavior or action affects your emotions.

But statements such as "I feel I am right," "You did it again," or "You don't understand," do not describe how you feel about an issue. They are your thoughts and opinions; they are perceived as judgmental and negative and result in defensive reactions from the other person. When this occurs the other person may no longer listen to you, but rather try to defend his or her position or action, which soon leads to a breakdown in communication. Thus, an important step is to identify your feelings first.

5. Express your feelings. State your feelings and emotions exactly the way you feel them and do not tone them down, make them nice, or pretend. This is very important. I have had to work on this one in particular, and although I have made some progress, I still have difficulty expressing my anger and resentment the way I should, due to my calm demeanor.

Expressing your feelings is very important, because that is the only way others know how you *really* feel. Certainly none of us wants to hurt the feelings of those close to us; but if they are not aware of how their actions affect our feelings, we leave ourselves open to more anger and frustration, as these same behaviors and actions will probably continue.

Expressing our feelings also helps relieve the tension that has been building inside us and leads to constructive problem-solving. This helps break the vicious cycle of attack, counterattack, and withdrawal that often arises when we allow tension and stress to build up until it erupts in angry confrontations.

My experience with identifying and expressing my feelings has been very constructive. It has certainly helped to improve communication between me and my wife and has led to a much closer marriage. It has also been quite helpful in my relationship with my parents.

For many years my parents, like many parents, treated me like a child and found fault with literally everything I said or did, despite the fact that I tried to be as respectful and accommodating toward them as possible. They did not like my low-fat diet, how I drove, and how I raised my children, just to name a few of their dislikes. Of course, after I learned about TMS I realized how their criticisms were really hurting me, making me angry and frustrated, but I had never told them how their constant criticism made me feel.

I have always tried to base my actions on reason and on knowledge from authoritative sources, so it really bothered me that instead of being respected by my parents I was ridiculed and chastised. Of course, most adults know that for many parents we remain their little children no matter how old we are. However, I remind my parents very politely that I am no longer five years old. I tell them that I respect them and love them, and that whatever I am doing is based on sound scientific knowledge and the many books I have read. I identify and express my feelings by letting them know how upsetting their comments are to me, and try to help them understand that they really hurt my feelings. This has helped to a great extent.

I also explain to them that the issue is not, for example, my diet, but rather respecting the life choices I have made as an informed adult. I also let them know that I find this manner of criticism degrading and unacceptable, especially when it is done in front of my wife and children, and that it is time for them to respect me for the respect I show them and to accept me as an adult.

My parents tell me that I am not the son they knew, and that I have changed. I certainly hope so! After the pain and disability I went through, I am glad to hear that I have made significant noticeable changes.

So identifying and expressing your feelings is a good beginning for establishing proper communication patterns between you and others.

6. Be specific, positive, and do not talk too much. Begin by saying something positive about the situation. Do not begin with negative statements such as, "You don't care about me." Be specific about how a particular phrase or behavior makes you feel.

For instance, you may feel that your spouse doesn't care about you because he or she often comes home late from work and is putting his or her career first, but you want to spend more time together. Instead of complaining about your spouse being late again, begin by expressing your feelings of loneliness and sadness. Explain how much you miss those nights when he or she gets home early and you get to spend more time together.

It is important to sum up what you want to say in three minutes or less. Talking longer than this may bore or frustrate the other person. Ask him or her for feedback or comments about what you said.

This is also a good time to ask the other party to repeat the main point of what you just said so that there will be no misunderstandings about what you are trying to convey. Make clear that you want this done in order to make certain that you have conveyed your concerns clearly. Otherwise, the other person might think you doubt his or her mental or hearing capabilities and be offended. This technique helps prevent misunderstandings and misinterpretations.

7. Never make assumptions; ask questions. After going through all the steps discussed so far, ask the other person why he or she said or did things in a way that hurt your feelings. Ask in an inquiring manner. For example, why he or she forgot to buy you a gift for that special occasion or to help you when you needed help. When faced with such an open and calm attitude, the other person feels that you are truly interested in communicating and not setting out to judge and condemn her or him.

Oftentimes we make incorrect assumptions and cause a great deal of anger and anxiety for ourselves and others, but by asking, and not judging, we save a great deal of misunderstanding and the problems that come with it. Of course, if you show willingness to work together so that such problems can be prevented in the future, then you can reach a much higher level of closeness in a relationship.

For example, when a husband says he forgot to remember that special occasion (again), what would happen if his wife said, "What do you think would help you remember?" and let him come up with a solution. This way he will remember it and be much more likely to follow through since it is his solution. Maybe he will suggest several calendars marked with important dates placed strategically in the bedroom, the bathroom, at work, and in the car to help him remember.

By trying to work out the problem together, instead of blaming each other while throwing in other points of disappointment and disagreement from the past, you can expect much better results. It is all about learning to work together to make the relationship better.

Another reason we should always ask questions and not make assumptions is because, as individuals with different backgrounds and different genders, there are times when we may judge circumstances based on certain assumptions, thinking of only one reason or explanation. However, our assumptions of why the other person looked, talked, or acted a certain way could be wrong and lead to misjudgment of the situation and/or the person. We may get very upset over what the other person said or did when they may have simply been trying to be helpful. This is why it is so important to ask and not make assumptions.

Deborah Tannen, in her book *You Just Don't Understand,* shares the results of her research into how men and women talk. A professor of linguistics at Georgetown University, she explains how gender differences in judging a situation can cause serious misunderstandings and hurt if one is not aware of these differences. The following passage from her book illustrates this point:

> Eve had a lump removed from her breast. Shortly after the operation, talking to her sister, she said that she found it upsetting to have been cut into, and that looking at the stitches was distressing because they left a seam that had changed the contour of her breast. Her sister said, "I know. When I had my operation I felt the same way." Eve made the same observation to her friend Karen, who said, "I know. It's like your body has been violated." But when she told her husband Mark how she felt, he said, "You can have plastic surgery to cover up the scar and restore the shape of your breast."
>
> Eve had been comforted by her sister and her friend, but she was not comforted by Mark's

comment. Quite the contrary, it upset her more. Not only didn't she hear what she wanted, that he understood her feelings, but, far worse, she felt he was asking her to undergo more surgery just when she was telling him how much this operation had upset her. "I'm not having anymore surgery!" she protested. "I'm sorry you don't like the way it looks." Mark was hurt and puzzled. "I don't care," he protested. "It doesn't bother me at all." She asked, "Then why are you telling me to have plastic surgery?" He answered, "Because *you* were upset about the way it looked." . . . Eve wanted the gift of understanding, but Mark gave her the gift of advice. He was taking the role of the problem solver, whereas she simply wanted confirmation of her feelings.[5]

Mark had been wonderfully supportive throughout Eve's surgery. However, like most men, he was solution oriented, so when she came to him with a problem, he said what naturally came to his mind. In this case Eve could have resolved the matter by expressing her feelings and saying, "I feel hurt by what you just said. Why did you say that?" or "I appreciate how supportive you have been, but what you just said really hurt me. Why did you say that?" This would have helped Mark to realize that he had inadvertently said something to upset her and, being the caring husband that he was, enabled him to find out why his advice hurt his wife's feelings. This could have helped both of them understand each others' needs and perspectives. But here they both felt hurt, and since they did not have a proper communication procedure in place, it got worse as they talked, until they decided to avoid the issue and stopped talking about it. Sound familiar?

This is exactly what my wife and I used to do before we improved our communication. She used to complain about her

---

[5] Tannen, Deborah, *You Just Don't Understand: Women and Men in Conversation* (New York: William Morrow and Company, 1990), pp. 49–50.

headache or backache and I would offer her advice instead of understanding and sympathy. She would get upset, assuming I did not care about her, but she kept her anger to herself. As a result she was sad and depressed around me, which in turn left me wondering what the problem was and made me upset. Of course, women's responses are also misunderstood by men and hurts *their* feelings. To quote Dr. Tannen again:

> If women are often frustrated because men do not respond to their troubles, men are often frustrated because women do. Some men not only take no comfort in such response they take offense. For example, a woman told me that when her companion talks about growing older, she responds, "I know how you feel; I feel the same way." To her surprise and chagrin, he gets annoyed; he feels she is trying to take something away from him by denying the uniqueness of his experience.
>
> A similar miscommunication was responsible for the following interchange, which began as a conversation and ended as an argument:
>
> He: I'm really tired. I didn't sleep well last night.
>
> She: I didn't sleep well either. I never do.
>
> He: Why are you trying to belittle me?
>
> She: I'm not! I'm just trying to show that I understand.[6]

This passage is another example of the kind of miscommunication my wife and I used to have that would upset me, and since I assumed she knew better than that, I used to get angry but kept my anger inside. Eventually, over several years, we reached a point where we stopped communicating completely. This meant that

---

[6] Tannen, p. 51. You may also consult Dr. John Gray's book *Men Are from Mars, Women Are from Venus* (New York: Harper Collins Publishers, 1992) for better understanding of how men and women can improve communication.

in many cases, unknowingly, we continued saying and doing things that upset and angered each other without realizing it.

Unfortunately, as in our case, many couples end up keeping the hurt to themselves. This hurt might remain with them for years, and as these feelings of hurt accumulate they may eventually manifest themselves as back pain or other disorders.

Thus, understanding some of these gender differences and subtleties can make a difference in how words and actions are perceived and judgments are formed. If we make an effort to learn and understand them, we can build better, stronger, and much more peaceful relationships with those close to us, especially our spouses. So always ask questions to help you understand and do not make assumptions.

Now It's Your Turn to Listen

8. Be a concerned, compassionate listener. If you want others to listen to your concerns and feelings with respect and understanding, you must do the same for them. As mentioned earlier, having mutual respect that allows you to share your concerns with your spouse, parents, or children and knowing that you will receive active, compassionate listening can do wonders to relieve stress and tension. This can lead to intimacy and greater closeness, even if the problem is difficult to solve. In marital and familial relationships it is extremely important to know that others do not take you for granted.

Have you ever just wanted to talk to someone about your problems and difficulties and found no one to listen, or felt that no one would be concerned enough to offer you understanding, strength, and encouragement? It is indeed a wonderful gift when your spouse and loved ones are also intimate friends with whom you can share your pain.

9. Acknowledge what the other person is saying. After listening actively and compassionately to the other person, let him or her know that you understand. You may not agree with the other person's perception of the situation, but your acknowledgment will show that you were listening and that you care. Simply repeating what they said by saying, "So you mean . . ." helps validate their feelings and concerns, although these might be contrary to yours. This will demonstrate your sincere desire to understand and be understood and will help you work together toward resolving the issues.

These strategies have made it easier for me to establish good communication and to prevent misunderstandings and the hurts that come with them. Practicing proper communication skills can help prevent misunderstandings, misjudgments, and hurt feelings and do wonders to improve relationships. This might not always be easy to do, especially when you are really hurt and upset, but if you practice these strategies often, they will become automatic, and not only prevent injuring the feelings of loved ones, but also lead to a more peaceful life.[7]

BUT I CAN'T DO THAT NOW

There are times, of course, when you can't communicate your feelings due to other pressing matters in your life. You or your loved one might be going through a personal crisis, or your work is causing you stress, and you have to wait for an appropriate time. So what can you do in such cases?

There are many strategies that can help you cope with tension and stress. These include breathing exercises, stretching, humor, gentle aerobic exercises such as swimming and walking, getting closer to nature, and others. My purpose for sharing these with you is to give you a summary of simple steps you can take to counter the effects of tension and stress on your mind and body and bring about a balance. Since I have a busy schedule, I have always tried to find

---

[7] I have to mention here that being kind, considerate, forgiving, and overlooking others' faults are essential components of a caring, respectful relationship. If you do not forgive and forget, but make an issue out of every little thing that bothers you, you will have difficulty establishing good communication based on mutual respect. Use good judgment and common sense, and do not allow your emotions and frustrations to get in the way.

those strategies and techniques that take little time to do, yet give good results.

I have included enough information here that you can reap the benefits of the stress-coping techniques discussed. However, I encourage you to learn more about these and other stress-coping methods through the available literature, some of which is listed in the bibliography, and apply those that fit your personality and lifestyle.

Now here are eleven coping strategies, many of which I use regularly, to help bring immediate or long-term relief.

ELEVEN COPING STRATEGIES

1. Breathing Exercises

When we experience any form of stress it is perceived as a threat, to which our bodies respond with what is known as the fight-or-flight response. The fight-or-flight response prepares our bodies to either run from the source of danger or fight it. However, in modern times the source of threat could be a stressful phone call, an angry boss, or an argument with your spouse. Your body may also respond in a similar way when you are angry over being stuck in a traffic jam or confronted with other daily aggravations.

Within the first six seconds of identifying the perceived threat our bodies go through the following emergency response:

1. Sympathetic nervous system activation; paying close attention to perceived threat
2. Tensing of muscles, especially facial muscles
3. Catching or holding breath or panting
4. Clenching jaws; constriction of blood flow to hands and feet.[8]

All of these changes occur very quickly. One effective way you can consciously counteract this response and bring your body back to its normal state is by practicing deep breathing.

---

[8] Stroebel, Charles, F. M.D., *QR: The Quieting Reflex (A Six Second Technique for Coping with Stress Anytime, Anywhere)* (New York: G. P. Putnam's Sons, 1982).

Your breathing pattern is one of the functions you should pay special attention to daily. If it is shallow and at chest level, not deep belly breathing, you can break this pattern by taking a deep breath that makes your belly expand, hold it for a few moments, and exhale slowly through your mouth. You may count to ten or say a word such as "relax" as you exhale. Repeat several times.

Why is it important to practice deep breathing? According to Dr. L. John Mayson, Ph.D.,

> Breathing properly is healthful; it increases the amount of oxygen in the blood, and strengthens weak abdominal and intestinal muscles. When you are tense or upset your breathing becomes shallow and irregular, and your heart rate tends to accelerate. When you are relaxed your breathing deepens and your heart rate decelerates. Breathing is the easiest physiological system to control. If you can breathe the deep, slow breath inherent in relaxation, then you can trigger the rest of the characteristics of the relaxation response. Once you become aware of your breathing patterns and know how to use breathing to reduce tension, you may gradually notice how you hold tension throughout your body.[9]

I have found the following breathing exercise, recommended by Anthony Robbins in *Unlimited Power,* quite helpful in reducing stress and tension and increasing my energy level:

> You should breathe in this ratio: inhale one count, hold four counts, exhale two counts. If you inhale for four seconds, you should hold for sixteen and exhale for eight. Why exhale twice as long as you inhale? That's when you eliminate toxins via your lymphatic system [which is the only way for your body's cells to drain off dead cells, toxins, and excess fluid]. Why hold four times as long? That's

---

[9] Mayson, L. John, Ph.D., *Guide to Stress Reduction* (Berkeley, Calif.: Celestial Arts, 1985), p. 14.

how you can fully oxygenate the blood and activate your lymphatic system. When you breathe, you should start from deep in your abdomen, like a vacuum cleaner that's getting rid of all toxins in the blood system.[10]

Robbins recommends that you take ten of these deep breaths three times a day, but do not strain yourself by inhaling or holding your breath for too long.

In addition to deep breathing to discharge stress and tension, I practice the progressive relaxation exercise mentioned as one of the mental exercises in Chapter Six. I have also discovered a very quick and effective means of countering the mental and physical effects of stress developed by Dr. Charles F. Stroebel, M.D., a professor of psychiatry at the University of Connecticut School of Medicine and lecturer at the Yale University School of Medicine. It is called the Quieting Reflex, or QR for short. He developed QR in his effort to find a cure for his own tension headaches after trying a number of relaxation techniques, including progressive relaxation and biofeedback.

QR has proven quite effective in treating patients with tension-related symptoms such as headaches and chronic back pain. It is also a very effective means of dealing with daily stresses as a gear-shifting technique that allows you to remain mentally alert while your body stays calm and less affected by the changes that occur due to stress. It aims at reversing your body's fight-or-flight response within the first six seconds and it works in the following manner:

1. Become aware of an annoyance, worry, or anxiety. If you don't sense one now, create tension by thrusting your tongue against the roof of your mouth for several seconds.
2. Smile inwardly with your mouth and eyes, and say to yourself, "Alert mind, calm body."
3. Inhale an easy, natural breath.

---

[10] Anthony Robbins, *Unlimited Power* (New York: Ballantine Books, 1986), pp. 169–172.

4. While exhaling, let your jaw, tongue, and shoulders go loose, feeling a wave of limpness, heaviness, and warmth flowing through your toes.

5. Resume normal activity. (For example, respond to the annoyance, but with an alert mind and a calm body. Was the worry worth a passing-gear response?) [11]

Watch your breathing pattern and try the exercises. These exercises not only help you counter many of the physical manifestations of tension but also make you more aware of your body's reaction to anger, anxiety, and tension. If your body responds to an annoyance or anxiety by tensing up your neck and/or shoulder muscles, you can immediately take action to relax them and avoid dealing with a stiff neck or shoulder pain.

The first place I experience tension is in my jaw joints. They become tense and tight when I am under stress or upset. Fortunately, by practicing these exercises I have developed enough awareness and sensitivity to my body's reaction to tension that I can recognize its early signs, practice QR, and prevent more severe manifestations of tension.

Remember that if you can recognize the early signs of stress response in your body and reverse it immediately, you can prevent it from accumulating and developing into chronic pain or serious health problems.

2. Stretch

In his book *Full Catastrophe Living: Using the Wisdom of Your Body and Mind to Face Stress, Pain, and Illness*, Jon Kabat-Zinn, Ph.D., founder and director of the Stress Reduction Clinic at the University of Massachusetts Medical Center, explains that after deep breathing, stretching tense muscles is the second technique to breaking the pattern of tension. He recommends a number of simple stretching exercises, including the back relaxer, shoulder rolls, neck

---

[11] Stroebel, p. 149.

rolls, and additional exercises to relax the major muscle groups.[12] You may consult his book for more detail.

3. Exercise

One benefit of regular aerobic exercise is that it works off tension and helps you cope better with stress. According to *The Complete Guide to Your Emotions and Your Health,*

> Every time you work out hard, you're helping to release pent-up tension. Immediately afterward, you'll feel relaxed, refreshed, and energized. As evidence of this, a study on fifteen men demonstrated that a 15-minute aerobic workout was sufficient to reduce anxiety below pre-exercise levels. Not only did tests show the men to be more relaxed immediately following their workout, but they remained that way twenty minutes later.[13]

Take advantage of the benefits of a regular aerobic exercise program, such as walking, jogging, or swimming to help you cope with tension. All you are trying to do is increase your heart rate by about 70 to 80 percent and oxygenate your body more efficiently. One way to gauge if you are doing it right is that you should sweat and still have enough breath to be able to talk a little. If you run out of breath, you are not doing it correctly. You may consult the books on health and fitness listed in the bibliography for more information on aerobic exercise.

I like the convenience of exercising at home and usually ski on my NordicTrack to get my aerobic exercise. One of the advantages of having an exercise machine at home is that even when I am very busy I can still get my daily aerobic exercise by hopping on the NordicTrack and exercising for ten to fifteen minutes.

---

[12] Kabat-Zinn, Jon, Ph.D., *Full Catastrophe Living: Using the Wisdom of Your Body and Mind to Face Stress, Pain, and Illness* (New York: Delacorte Press, 1990).

[13] Padus, Emrika, *The Complete Guide to Your Emotions and Your Health* (Emmaus, Pa.: Rodale Press, 1992), p. 23.

Nowadays, I have reached a point where I can ski with my eyes closed and not lose my balance. This allows me to practice visualization while skiing. I close my eyes and see myself skiing Yosemite National Park in winter. I feel the cold crisp air around me and the warmth of sun on my face. I breathe in the fresh air and see the beauty of snow-covered scenery. Then I travel to different cities and countries and visit many fascinating people and places while skiing on my NordicTrack. It is a wonderful, relaxing experience that not only provides me, with a chance to improve my ability to visualize, but also gives me a mental vacation from the stresses of daily life.

4. Humor Helps

Humor can also play an important role in reducing tension and improving health. According to *The Complete Guide to Your Emotions and Your Health*,

> The stress-relieving power of humor is well established. Laughter, we are told, relieves tension, breaks negative "holding patterns," and helps put our problems in perspective. In fact, a study of mid-life wellness factors by Harvard's eminent George Vaillant, M.D., singled out humor as a major stress-coping mechanism among healthy men. No small wonder then that humor has been credited with reducing the coronary risk of a high-stress lifestyle.[14]

In his book *Anatomy of an Illness* (Norton, 1979), Norman Cousins described how through laughter he was able to overcome his crippling condition. His account was first published in the *New England Journal of Medicine* (December 1976) and later led to his becoming an adjunct professor at the UCLA School of Medicine. In fact, through laughter, Norman Cousins was able to reduce and later eliminate his need for pain medications, and eventually prove the specialists wrong and recover. I highly recommend reading *Anatomy*

---

[14] Padus, p. 543.

of an Illness as a testimony to the interaction between our emotions and health.

Humor serves to lessen the mental and physical effects of stress. It helps us focus on the positive side and think more clearly in dealing with problems. If we are overwhelmed and depressed by problems and difficulties, we will be less efficient in dealing with them. Keeping a sense of humor, whether you are caught in a traffic jam or a client got on your nerves, can be quite an asset in coping with stress and tension.

5. Nutrition

A healthy diet also plays an important role in the way we feel and our ability to handle stress and tension. After researching what constitutes a healthy diet and considering the many contradictory opinions that exist among the experts, I came to the conclusion that moderation is the answer. I think we have to look at how our individual bodies react to different foods and consider those effects on our emotions as one factor in reducing tension and stress.

Too much caffeine and stress do not mix. Smoking and drinking don't help the situation, either. A healthy diet of fruits, vegetables, grains, and legumes that is high in carbohydrates and low in fat; daily vitamins and minerals; and occasional consumption of fish, chicken, and lean meat helps me keep up with my daily activities and handle stress better. I avoid eating processed foods as much as possible due to their high sodium, fat, and sugar content in addition to the preservatives and other chemicals that are added to them.

In times of stress and tension I also avoid heavy meals and follow Dr. Judith Wurtman's advice. In her book, *Managing Your Mind and Mood Through Food*, Dr. Wurtman, a research scientist at Massachusetts Institute of Technology, recommends a high-carbohydrate, low-fat diet for dealing with severe to mild stress. Her research has demonstrated that:

> . . . in a stressed state the brain more quickly uses up its supply of the chemicals that dictate emotions and state of mind. When the brain begins to make more serotonin [the calming chemical], as it

does when carbohydrates are eaten, negative feelings are eased; anger is moderate, worrisome problems seem to shrink in magnitude, the edge is taken off anxiety, tension diminishes, and it becomes easier to deal with frustration.

Eating carbohydrates takes the immediate pressure off long enough to enable you to stand back and consider more rationally and coolly the options for dealing with the cause of your stress.[15]

She recommends about two ounces of pure carbohydrates, such as a bagel, twelve crackers, or two ounces of oatmeal without milk. And if you are too stressed out to eat, sip a cup of sweetened herb tea with sugar or honey, or drink eight ounces of caffeine-free soft drink. To maximize the calming benefits of carbohydrates, she recommends eating or drinking them slowly and under an enjoyable condition or while staring out the window. I would also suggest taking a deep breath and letting all the tension out of your system before you eat. It does make a difference.

The following quote from Dr. Edward E. Rosenbaum's *A Taste of My Own Medicine* sums up my overall feelings about nutrition and diet in general:

I am convinced that there is no simple best diet for everyone. There are too many genetic differences between people. Some can handle fats, some can't; some thrive on milk, some don't; and some can handle candy, though a diabetic can't.

The statistics we have today seem to show that the lean do better than the fat, that a low-cholesterol, high-roughage diet makes sense. That's my opinion at this writing, but to generalize on diet is like giving the same pill to all people for all illnesses. And I've seen the statistics change a few times in my time.[16]

[15] Wurtman, Judith, J., Ph.D. *Managing Your Mind and Mood Through Food* (New York: HarperCollins, 1987), p. 230.

[16] Rosenbaum, Edward, E., M.D., *A Taste of My Own Medicine* (New York: Random House, 1988), p. 82. In this book Dr. Rosenbaum, a

6. Stop and Smell the Roses

Give yourself a break. Take a day off from work or arrange for babysitting and give yourself a chance to rest and get away from it all and get close to nature, even for an hour or two. Take time to smell the roses, literally. Go to a park or a flower garden or hike a trail. Get close to nature and leave your worries behind for a little while.

Many studies have shown that being in a natural environment, or even looking at pictures or videotapes of nature, help people recuperate better from stress. You may consider mounting posters of mountains and trees on your walls at home or at work, or have live plants to look at. Simply looking at nature's beauty has such a positive impact on human mind and body that ". . . Surgery patients recovered faster if they had bedside windows that looked out on nature, as opposed to windows that fronted a brick wall."[17] And patients in whose rooms posters of water and trees were mounted reported less anxiety, required fewer doses of pain-killing medication, and recovered faster than patients who were exposed to abstract pictures, white panels, or no pictures, according to research at Texas A&M University.[18] So take advantage of these benefits and get closer to nature.

If you can manage to go on a weekend getaway or a vacation to the lake or the mountains, do it. Going away from your troubles and responsibilities will not only help relax you, but it may also help you think more clearly and find a solution to your problems.

---

professor at Oregon Health Sciences University, recounts his experiences as a cancer patient and the many difficulties he faced with the medical system. I have to mention here that I do take vitamin supplements daily, such as 1000 mg of vitamin C, and try to rely more on natural and herbal treatments than manufactured drugs. However, if I have an ear infection, I rush to my doctor to get antibiotics. There are limits to the effectiveness of any treatment, so I try to take the middle path and incorporate the best of each discipline into what works best for me.

[17] Faelton, Sharon, and David Diamond, *Tension Turnaround* (Emmaus, Pa.: Rodale Press, 1990), p. 169.

[18] *Health Confidential*, Boardroom Inc., May 1995, p. 15.

7. Scramble Negative Thoughts

If negative thoughts keep running through your head and causing you stress and tension, and you find it difficult to stop them, try scrambling them! Anthony Robbins recommends changing the negative sensations we link to a distressing thought pattern into positive sensations, so they lose their negative impact. The following technique is from his book *Awaken the Giant Within*:

> A simple way of breaking a pattern is by **scrambling the sensations** we link to our memories. The only reason we're upset is that we're representing things in a certain way in our minds. For example, if your boss yells at you, and you mentally rerun that experience the rest of the day, picturing him or her yelling at you over and over again, then you'll feel progressively worse. Why let the experience continue to affect you? Why not take the record in your mind and scratch it so many times that you can't experience those feelings anymore? Maybe you can make it funny!

He suggests scrambling these images by closing your eyes and, with a big grin on your face, seeing the entire incident as a movie. Then turn it into a cartoon; see people swallowing their words, growing funny noses and ears. Run it fast forwards and backwards. Do so many crazy things to it that pretty soon you begin to laugh when you think of that incident and it no longer bothers you.

I have tried a variation of this technique and found it quite useful. Once, after being insulted by the owner of a food facility upon completion of an inspection, I left the facility quite angry and upset. I decided this was a good time to give this technique a try. I sat in my car, reclined the seat, and with a big smile on my face, I imagined the owner who had offended me playing the part of a clown in a funny movie. I saw him dressed as a clown, slipping and falling over and over again, and unable to gain his balance. I saw bubbles coming out of his mouth every time he tried to speak; the bubbles burst on his face, making him all soapy. After doing this several times, all my anger came out as laughter. I laughed every time I remembered that incident for the rest of the day. A day that could have been ruined because of him turned into a nice one after all.

Do whatever you can to break these patterns as soon as possible so that such incidents do not occupy your mind and exhaust your energies. You can also perform certain acts, such as jumping up in the air and shouting, "I feel great," several times to break the pattern of negative thoughts; or ask yourself nonsensical trivia questions that distract your mind and keep it busy, such as, "How many ants can I fit on a spoon?" or "How long will it take to read a million pages?"

Have you noticed how you can be absorbed in your thoughts or a conversation when someone distracts you by asking a question? And then, after thinking about the question, you cannot remember what you were saying or thinking about before? It is the same principle, except that you are doing it for yourself.[19]

8. Change Your Focus, Think Positive

Sometimes we get so focused on a problem that we are unable to see the solution even when it stares us in the face. It helps to look at problems from different perspectives. By focusing on some of the positive aspects of a situation, you might be able to deal with it in a more constructive fashion. This may help you cope with tension and stress by reducing your fears and worries.

I try to look at every situation as a learning experience and find the positive side of it. During months of pain and disability, I tried to keep my mind focused on the big picture, hoping that by learning more and more about my condition I might help others to avoid suffering the same way. I am glad I took that approach, because it helped me continue with my search for an answer.

In matters such as relationship difficulties, where other people are involved, we sometimes get impatient and lose sight of the positive side of the relationship, causing ourselves more agony and pain than is really there. Try to take some time out from the usual patterns of

---

[19] For complete details of these and other techniques, see *Awaken the Giant Within* by Anthony Robbins (New York: Fireside, 1992).

conflict and withdrawal to focus on positive aspects and take a different approach or try a new perspective.

9. Write It Down

In a study conducted at Southern Methodist University, twenty-five students were asked to write for twenty minutes a day for four days about problem situations they had been unable to resolve. Another group of twenty-five students wrote for the same time period, but wrote about trivial topics.

Blood samples taken before and just after the experiment, as well as six weeks later, showed that students who wrote out their negative feelings had an increased immune (T-cell) response. The second group of students showed no such improvement.

A similar experiment with another group of students revealed that "students who documented their stress about coming to college had significantly fewer health problems, and remained healthier up to five months later, than those who wrote about trivial things."[20]

Clearly, expressing negative feelings, even in writing, can help not only to make us feel better by getting it out of our systems, but also it can have positive effects on our health. So try to make time for about twenty minutes a day to write about matters that bother you and cause tension.

If you are too busy to do this, at least write an outline. You can do it in your car before getting home, during your lunch break, or any other time that you have a few minutes to yourself without interruptions.

10. Go Heart-to-Heart with God

Many years ago, when I set out to establish empowering beliefs and principles that would enhance the quality of my life, I found many studies that pointed out how people with a strong belief in a loving and just creator lived happier and healthier lives. The

---

[20] Michaud, Ellen, and Alice Feinstein, *Prevention Magazine's 30-Day Immune Power Program* (Emmaus, Pa.: Rodale Books, 1992), pp. 196–197.

psychological benefits of knowing that I was not just an accident whose life might end at any moment by another accident, and that I was watched and cared for by The One who created all things, was certainly good enough reason to believe in God.

However, observing the order in the universe and the natural wonders within us and all around us, and experiencing the effectiveness of prayers, helped make belief in God an essential aspect of a comprehensive life program.

Interestingly enough, Dr. Larry Dossey, M.D., cites a number of studies in his book *Healing Words: The Power of Prayer and the Practice of Medicine* in which prayed-for patients did better than those not prayed for. In one such case a randomized, double blind study of 393 heart patients revealed that the prayed-for patients were five times less likely to require antibiotics and three times less likely to develop pulmonary edema (fluid in the lungs). Also, none of the prayed-for patients required endotracheal intubalation, in which an airway is inserted in the trachea attached to a mechanical ventilator, while 6 percent of the patients in the other group required it. Commenting on this study Dr. Dossey writes, "If the technique being studied had been a new drug or a surgical procedure instead of prayer, it would almost certainly have been heralded as some sort of 'breakthrough.'"[21]

Dr. Dossey points out that medicine does not need to understand how prayer works, the same way that it does not know exactly how certain medications work, but that as long as there is scientific proof that prayer is effective, it must be considered as one more option in enhancing patients' treatment.

The point of all this is that it certainly pays to believe in God and pray to him. Consider setting aside a particular time, maybe late at night when everyone is asleep, or early morning, and have a heart-to-heart talk with your creator. You can tell him about everything that bothers you and ask him, with confidence and certainty, for relief, patience, guidance, help, and peace.

---

[21] Dossey, Larry, M.D. *Healing Words: The Power of Prayer and the Practice of Medicine* (San Francisco: Harper San Francisco, 1993), p. 180.

If you have not done this before, it may feel strange at first, but you will be amazed how peaceful and light you feel after a few sessions; and if what you are asking is for your ultimate good, it might be granted to you sooner than you expect it. Don't hold anything back, because He knows and sees all things and truly cares.

11. Count Your Blessings

As an addendum to the above strategy, you might also count your blessings while you are having your heart-to-heart talk with God. Sometimes, when we get caught in negative thought patterns and as our problems seem to get constantly worse, we lose sight of the many positive things in our lives. Spending a few minutes to count our blessings and feel grateful for them can improve our emotional state fairly quickly.

I usually begin with parts of my body and the many faculties and capabilities I have been blessed with. I thank God for my eyes, ears, mouth, hands, and so on, and continue till I reach my toes. I also thank Him for having normal internal organs such as healthy lungs, heart, liver, and kidneys. Then I take a deep breath, feeling the air going through my entire body.

I feel grateful for the many things I can do daily because I have been given these blessings and realize how difficult my life would have been if any part of my body was missing, in pain, or not functioning properly. If this is done regularly with a deep feeling of appreciation and gratitude, it helps reduce anxiety and tension.

Just imagine how your life would have been if in addition to all the stress and tension you have, you had a physical problem too. Actually, if you suffer or have suffered from chronic pain and disability, you know exactly what I mean.

But our countless blessings are not limited to our minds and bodies. The air we breathe, the food we eat, and the water we drink help us sustain ourselves and without them we would perish. These are all blessings to be grateful for. Taking a few moments every day to count our blessings and show gratitude for them will help us put matters in a better perspective. It certainly helps me, for I know that there is always someone else in worse condition than I am.

These are some of the strategies I use and that you might try to cope with a difficult situation that causes you stress and tension. You may also refer to some of the books on mind/body connection in the bibliography for additional resources.

A word of caution, though, these are coping strategies, not avoidance strategies. They are meant to help you reduce tension until you can resolve stressful issues through proper communication and cooperation. Do not use these strategies to create a comfort zone and avoid resolving the underlying problems that are the real source of tension. If you do, you leave yourself vulnerable to TMS and other disorders.

WELL, ABOUT TIME!

Finally, you find the right time to communicate your feelings and concerns. Using the strategies mentioned earlier in this chapter, you may find the other person more receptive than before, and you will be on your way to a better relationship. These strategies have worked very well for me so far and have brought about better understanding and a stronger relationship with my wife and others.

However, what do you do when your communication efforts do not produce the expected results? You may find the other party has had so many bad experiences that your voice is not heard and your concerns are neglected. So what can you do now? Sometimes you need to wait and try again, perhaps several times, until the other party believes you are sincere and committed to communicating and improving the situation. However, sometimes a third party must be brought in to help you open the lines of communication.

If the person you need to communicate with is your spouse and you have difficulty resolving the issues together, it may be wise to get an impartial third person or a family counselor to mediate the situation. In this case, as in other situations, I believe the best way to solve any problem, medical or personal, is to seek those methods and solutions that utilize and foster our innate capabilities and potentials. That is why I highly recommend Michele Weiner-Davis's book *Divorce Busting: A Revolutionary and Rapid Program for Staying Together.*

Divorce Busting is a solution-oriented book that can help resolve many marital conflicts and bring peace and harmony. You do not have to be at the brink of divorce to read it or use its methods.

Based on the author's many years of experience as a therapist, this book teaches Solution-Oriented Brief Therapy (SBT). Unlike therapists who spend many months trying to find the psychological and emotional reasons underlying behaviors and conflicts, this method concentrates on resolving issues and behaviors that cause the problem and works to modify them into a solution that will create harmony between the couple.

Psychodynamic therapy is based on the idea that only a trained eye can perceive the so-called *real* problem, therefore, as a lay person describes the symptom, the supposed expert ascertains the goal of treatment. SBT is not founded on this premise. We believe that people know themselves best and that they are the experts on what needs to change, not the therapist. So when therapy begins, clients are asked, "What is it that you would like to change?" and this is the starting point in therapy.[22]

In fact, the author notes that two-thirds of her clients reported improvement in their relationships prior to their first counseling appointments, which demonstrates that couples have the resources to resolve their own problems, once they decide to use them. The therapist simply facilitates the process by building on strengths rather than dissecting weaknesses. Appropriately enough, she has a sign posted in her office that reads, "Please solve your problems in advance so I can help you more."

Weiner-Davis offers many valuable ideas, solutions, and strategies to improve relationships throughout *Divorce Busting*. However, to resolve conflicts and improve a marriage immediately, there are four basic steps you must take to make desirable behaviors grow:

---

[22] Weiner-Davis, Michele, *Divorce Busting: A Revolutionary and Rapid Program for Staying Together* (New York: Summit Books, 1992), p. 89.

1. Step 1: Describe as clearly and specifically as possible what troubles you about your spouse and/or your marriage.
2. Step 2: Identify the exceptions—times when the problem doesn't occur, when it is less frequent, shorter duration, less intense or not as annoying.
3. Step 3: Determine your role in making the exceptions happen.
4. Step 4: Repeat what has worked. [23]

The author advises you to think about these steps and write down your responses to help clarify your thoughts. Identify those instances when the relationship has been at its best and repeat the actions and behaviors that have worked.

You should also try to do less of the things that do not work. For example, if you complain to your husband about him not being affectionate and he does not become more caring and loving, but when you put on make-up or cook his favorite meal he does become more affectionate, that's your answer. You might wonder, with all the problems and responsibilities you have to deal with, when you will have time to do this. Certainly a reasonable husband does not expect this every day; however, if putting on some make-up has worked in the past to make your husband more affectionate, then do more of that and less complaining.

Of course, the same applies to the husband. Has helping out around the house or taking your wife out to dinner worked in the past? Then do it.

Doing what works means that even if you feel that you should not have to do it, you will do it because it helps to harmonize the marriage (as long as it does not involve anything illegal or immoral—use good judgment).

Weiner-Davis offers many useful strategies for getting results within a month, even if you use them alone, by focusing on solutions, not problems. She also has advice on how to interrupt destructive patterns, establish new patterns that work, and keep the positive

---

[23] Weiner-Davis, p. 140.

changes going.She offers a few more strategies and solutions that you may want to read on your own and apply according to your needs and circumstances.

A recent study conducted by Dr. John Gottman and published in *Psychology Today*, titled "What Makes Marriages Work," revealed that the happiest marriages are those in which there are more positive feelings and interactions than negative ones.

> Across the board I found there was a very specific ratio that exists between the amount of positivity and negativity in a stable marriage. . . . That magic number is 5 to 1. As long as there is five times as much positive feelings and interaction between husband and wife as there is negative, the marriage was likely to be stable over time. In contrast, those couples who were heading for divorce were doing far too little on the positive side to compensate for the growing negativity between them.[24]

Dr. Gottman states that this was true of all three types of marriage: validating marriages in which couples compromise often and calmly work out their problems to mutual satisfaction as they arise; volatile marriages in which conflicts erupt often and result in passionate disputes; and conflict-avoiding in which couples agree to disagree, rarely confronting their differences head-on. So try to create more positivity in your marriage by being kind and caring to your spouse and by creating special moments and memories that last, on a regular basis.

Certainly in every marriage there are times when passionate discussions, arguments, or conflicts occur, but having more positivity helps to keep things in perspective and keep the relationship strong.

---

[24] Gottman, John, "What Makes Marriages Work," *Psychology Today* (March/April 1994), p. 41.

THE ONE MINUTE FAMILY

Raising children is a great responsibility and a challenging task. It can be a major source of anxiety and tension. I had always dreamt of providing my children with a loving and caring atmosphere. I wanted to give them a family life that built their self-esteem and self-confidence and prepared them for the challenges and responsibilities of adulthood. So I always look for information on parenting and better ways of raising children.

Many books are written on this subject on the best ways to raise children. Here too I believe the methods and strategies that utilize the child's own resources work best. Such strategies help build self-confidence and self-esteem and allow the children to make their own decisions from an early age and be responsible for the consequences of those decisions. Children who are allowed to make their own decisions and experience the negative or positive consequences of those decisions will become much better decision makers later in life.

Allowing children to be more responsible for their decisions and actions involves them directly in their own upbringing and takes a great deal of the burden off the parents. It also makes it difficult for them to disobey and rebel against the rules; after all, they set the rules themselves.

If you are wondering how this can be done, it is easier than you think. Dr. Spencer Johnson, known as the coauthor of *The One Minute Manager*, is the author of two books on parenthood, *The One Minute Father* and *The One Minute Mother*. In his two books on parenting he has applied what has worked best in managing companies to raising a family. It works because those management principles are based on what works best with human nature. One Minute Parenting consists of three steps:

1. One Minute Goals
2. One Minute Praisings
3. One Minute Reprimands

One Minute Goals

In any organization, clear rules and goals help individuals know exactly what is expected of them and facilitates accomplishment of their tasks. Unfortunately, in many families, since children are not involved in the decision-making process, they do not feel obligated to follow the rules.

In this method, rules and goals are not set by the parents alone. Rather they are agreed upon in a family meeting where everyone participates and helps in the decision making, even the youngest family members. If you wonder whether that this could mean more problems, since children probably want to set easy rules, you could be in for a big surprise.

Once we had a family meeting about watching television. It was the end of the summer vacation, and as parents we thought it would be better if our daughter and son watched less television. After we all presented our opinions and discussed the advantages and disadvantages of each one, my son, who was five years old then, suggested no TV during the week, one hour on Friday night, two hours on Saturday, and one hour on Sunday.

My daughter, seven years old at the time, suggested that if they did all their homework and had been good on any day, they should get to watch television that day.

Their mother and I felt the less TV the better, and sided with our son. So the first suggestion was approved 3-1. We did agree, however, to review this rule in future family meetings.

I am happy to report that the kids have lived up to the goal of watching a total of four hours of television for the entire week. They spend more time playing, inventing new games, reading books, improving their gymnastics and karate skills, and engaging in more fruitful activities than watching television. In fact, they monitor themselves and turn the television off at the end of the hour without any need for us to remind them or use parental power. It's a win-win situation.

I mention this incident to show that in most cases children are quite aware of what is good for them, and when given the opportunity to be responsible for their decisions and actions, they can be even stricter on themselves than adults.

Of course, common sense dictates that not all issues be left to the children's discretion. On issues of healthy and safety we set the rules, even if they do not agree, but explain to them the reasons why. For example, if they refuse to take a certain medication because they do not like its taste, we give it to them regardless. However, many issues can be resolved more easily and to the satisfaction of both parents and kids if children play a role in setting the rules and goals.

Why are they called One Minute Goals? Because they are less than 250 words and take about one minute to read them off the paper. If it takes less than a minute that is fine, but any longer than that means you have too many goals and it might be difficult to achieve them. When this happens, it leads to negative feelings of failure and disappointment, which makes the process ineffective.

Prior to becoming a One Minute Family, my wife and I had tried the reward system in order to encourage our children to keep their rooms clean, make their beds, go to karate class, etc. It was successful for the most part; however, I had always felt uncomfortable about giving them a reward for what they should consider their responsibility and duty.

My wife and I certainly do not get a reward for washing the dishes or making our bed, and many duties and responsibilities, such as parenting, must be done properly, while there are no material rewards. The reward method set an expectation that for every good deed there must be some material reward, and this is simply not the case in the real world.

In her book on parenting, Barbara Coloroso, an internationally recognized speaker on parenting, writes the following about the reward system:

> Kids who are consistently bribed and rewarded are likely to grow into adults who are overly dependent on others for approval and recognition, lacking their own self-confidence and sense of responsibility. The questions they will often ask are:
> * What's in it for me?

- What's the payoff?
- Does it count for anything?
- Do you like it?
- Did you see me do it?
- Did I do it right?[25]

When we had our first family meeting, we decided to set goals in three areas: chores, rules, and things to do. I asked, "How do we want our home to look?" and let everyone come up with an answer. This led to the following three chores: keep the shoes in the closet, the rooms clean, and make the beds in the morning.

For the rules category, we concentrated on things that helped us cooperate better. So the rules were sharing, listening, and no fighting.

For things to do during the week we had to negotiate an agreement. One concern was going to karate classes regularly. Although our children enjoyed karate when they got to class, they took a long time to get ready and most of the time preferred to stay home and play instead. Some days it took my wife more than half an hour to get them ready to go, by the end of which she was frustrated and exhausted.

My wife wanted the children to attend karate classes four times a week, but they wanted to go only once a week. After some intense negotiation we all agreed on going to karate three times a week. Once they made the commitment my wife has had very little difficulty getting them ready (well, most of the time!). The children also agreed to get their homework done, and do one good thing for each other every day.

Of course, mom and dad also set similar goals. After all, parents must set good examples and they too are part of the family team.

Once the goals were set and written down (in my son's case, drawn), we reviewed them, posted them somewhere visible, and reviewed them regularly so that they became a part of us. We also turned goal reviewing into a game by asking who could name the first

---

[25] Coloroso, Barbara, *Kids Are Worth it! Giving Your Child the Gift of Inner Discipline* (New York: William Morrow & Company, 1994), p. 19.

chore or the second rule as we drove to school or other places. In my experience the more the goal is reviewed, the more it becomes a part of our subconscious behavior, a habit, and a natural thing to do.

I was amazed how effective these goals were when next day my son and daughter shared a toy instead of arguing over it. They were so nice to each other that it was unreal. This does not mean that they have never argued since, but it helped to keep them doing more good things for each other and reduced sibling rivalry.

Setting One Minute Goals consists of the following components:

1. To have clear goals as a family and as individuals.
2. To reach mutual agreements so everyone feels he or she is an important member of the family.
3. Each person writes out the goals in 250 words or less on a single piece of paper, so it takes only a minute or so to reread them.
4. The goals are specific, showing exactly what we would each like to see happen and when.
5. Goals are reread and reviewed often in order to make them mental habits, a way of thinking.
6. Parents examine the children for a minute or so at frequent intervals (more often at the beginning) to see if their behavior matches their goals.
7. Once a week, the goals are reviewed in a family meeting.[26]

This is a guideline, and you can certainly use your creativity in this matter. One thing we do is rotate the responsibility of running the meeting each time. In this way the children learn what it means to be a leader. It builds their self-confidence and self-esteem and prepares them for the future.

I try to associate these meetings with as much positivity as possible by bringing popcorn or other refreshments and playing games after the meeting.

---

[26] Adapted from *The One Minute Father* by Dr. Spencer Johnson, M.D. (New York: William Morrow and Company, 1983), p. 59.

One Minute Praising

This is the second step. As you might have already guessed, it takes about a minute to do and is quite easy. How does it work? In the words of Dr. Johnson,

One Minute Praisings work well when:

1. I tell my children ahead of time that I am going to praise them when they do something that makes me feel good. And I encourage them to do the same with me.
2. I catch my children doing something *right*.
3. I tell my children specifically what they did.
4. Then I tell them how good I *feel* about what they did and why it makes me feel so good.
5. I stop talking for a few seconds. The silence lets *them* feel the good feelings themselves.
6. Then I tell them that I *love* them.
7. I end the praising with a *hug* or at least a light touch to let them know I care.
8. The praising is short and sweet. When it's over, it's over.
9. I realized that it takes me only a minute to praise my children. But feeling good about themselves may last *them* for a lifetime.
10. I know that what I am doing is good for my children *and* for me. I feel really good about *myself.*[27]

When you review the goals during the meeting, or any time you notice your children are getting closer to achieving their goals, you call them and give them a One Minute Praising.

This simple yet very effective method lets them know that their efforts are noticed and appreciated, and the good feelings it gives them encourages them to do even more good. In my house, we even give each other high tens to put more action into it. Kids love it. They ask me to hold my hands high so they can jump really high when they want to give me a high ten. These praisings need not be restricted only

---

[27] Johnson, p. 48.

to achieving One Minute Goals. For instance, on those occasions when kids join me for grocery shopping we do it as a team and give each other high tens for excellent teamwork.

The One Minute Praisings leave us all feeling closer and let us hug and express our love to each other several times a day. As I mentioned, we have added high tens to the process, and you might want to come up with a few innovations of your own, depending on your children's age and your lifestyle.

One Minute Reprimands

After several weeks when the children have shown real improvement in achieving their One Minute Goals and have received One Minute Praisings, you may need to use One Minute Reprimands to deal with misbehavior and lack of progress.

This is similar to One Minute Praisings, except that in this case, you first tell the children that you are going to use a new way of disciplining them. Again in the words of Dr. Johnson,

> The One Minute Reprimand works well when:
>
> 1. I tell my children beforehand that I am going to reprimand them when their behavior is unacceptable to me. And I encourage them to be just as honest to me.
> **The First Half of the Reprimand**
> 2. I reprimand my children as soon as possible.
> 3. I tell them *specifically* what they did.
> 4. I tell my children, in no uncertain terms, just how I *feel* about what they have done.
> 5. I am silent for a few very long, unpleasant seconds to let them *feel* what I feel.
> **The Second Half of the Reprimand**
> 6. Then I calm down and *touch* my children in a way that lets them know that I am on their side.
> 7. I remind my children that while their recent behavior was not good, I think *they* are good.

8. I tell my children, "I love you!" and I hug them. When the reprimand is over, it's over. I don't mention it again.

9. Later in the day, I listen to whatever the children want to tell me.

10. I realize that while it may take me only a minute to reprimand my children with love, the benefits may last for a *lifetime.*[28]

Instead of grounding them or taking away privileges, you let your children know exactly what they did wrong and how angry it makes you feel (remember this is feeling, so express it as feelings in your tone of voice and facial expressions). Wait a few seconds and let the child feel your anger, then tell the child how much you love him or her and that you believe she or he can do better than that.

While the One Minute Reprimand makes children feel chastised and punished, it makes it clear that although their behavior made you angry, you still love them and you believe they have the ability to exhibit better behavior than that. They are left feeling that their behavior was bad, not them, that they have their parents' love and confidence, and that they can do better. In fact, they can give themselves a One Minute Reprimand when they do not achieve their goals or behave well. And they do! You might consider trying it on yourself as well when you get lazy and don't achieve your goals.

We have tried to be a One Minute Family for the past few months, and I have to say that it has worked very well. The only secret is doing it. Setting aside fifteen or twenty minutes a week for a family meeting, reviewing the goals during the week, and the other steps take very little time; however, being a new technique, it may take some planning and getting used to.

Unfortunately, in most cases there is never enough time for the important things, but we can always make time for urgent matters. There is not enough time to have a family meeting and set goals in order to prevent problems, but there is always time to discipline the children for not making their beds or for constantly fighting. Isn't that

---

[28] Johnson, p. 24.

usually the case? But if you make a serious commitment to put these strategies into practice, you will see good results. [29]

Whenever we get too busy to have our family meetings, we begin to feel the effects of it and return to our meetings and One Minute Goals immediately.

We also use some of the techniques offered by Barbara Coloroso in her book *Kids Are Worth It!* The crux of her arguments and strategies is empowering children by teaching them how to think and resolve their problems, instead of simply being told by their parents what to think and do.

Empowering our children involves first giving them a secure, safe, nurturing environment offering them unconditional love, caring touch, tenderness, and concern for their physical, emotional, and spiritual well-being. With a strong, loving foundation in place we can begin to give our children the opportunity to make choices and decisions, all the while providing a structure on which they can build, increasing their responsibilities and decision-making opportunities as they grow. Teaching them to make their own decisions enables them to learn to be responsible for themselves, and exercise their own rights while respecting the rights and legitimate needs of others.

If we accept that we can influence and empower our children, we will no longer feel that we must control them and make them mind. We can then begin to look at the empowerment tools that are the alternatives to the manipulative tools of

---

[29] If you are experiencing difficulty with managing your time, as most of us do, I highly recommend Dr. Stephen R. Covey's book *First Things First* (New York: Simon & Shuster, 1994). He is the chairman and founder of Covey Leadership Center and author of several books, including *The 7 Habits of Highly Effective People.*

behavioral management. They are encouragement [not rewards] and discipline [not punishment].[30]

I have given a brief summary of the techniques explained in *The One Minute Father* or *The One Minute Mother*. I recommend reading them as well as *Kids Are Worth It!* in order to fully understand the concepts and techniques and their benefits.

IS IT PERFECT YET?

These techniques and strategies in communication and child rearing have helped to bring about many wonderful changes in my life and the life of my family. But anyone who is married and has children knows about the challenges involved. As family therapist Michele Weiner-Davis puts it:

> When I was pregnant with my first child, my husband and I attended a series of Lamaze classes. In preparation for parenthood, one of the last classes was devoted to life with children. I distinctly remember my instructor's solution to the fatigue she felt from the never-ending demands of her three children. She confessed that she would lock herself in her room for five minutes, telling her children that her room was off-limits. She would fall into a Zen-like meditative state, then reappear downstairs refreshed. My reaction to her parenting tip was so extreme, I couldn't wait for the class to end to hear my husband's response. I almost laughed out loud when she told us that five minutes did the trick for her. "Here is a woman who is obviously satisfied with very little," I thought to myself. "She thinks that stealing away for five short minutes is a major accomplishment. She's either a martyr or some extreme version of supermom." As we walked to our car (should I say waddled), my husband said he

---

[30] Coloroso, p. 26. *Health* (Emmaus, Pa.: Rodale Press, 1992), p. 23.

agreed with me completely. We shook our heads and laughed all the way home.

We are not laughing anymore. Now, some ten parenting years and two children later, our eyes have been opened. What I wouldn't give for five (even three) minutes of solitude on our many frenzied days. We obviously had a great deal to learn about children and being parents. Needless to say, our many erroneous and idealistic expectations about raising children made the transition into parenthood a challenging one.[31]

No, things are not perfect. Many of my idealistic expectations about marriage and parenthood have not come true. My kids don't always behave the way I like them to, especially in front of others; occasionally my wife and I have an argument or two; but that just about makes us a typical, normal family and human beings. I feel because of what I went through I have grown in many ways and see things in a better light, and, most importantly, learned to live with my and others' imperfections.

These are some of the strategies and techniques that have helped me improve those aspects of my life that were constant sources of tension and stress. I am very fortunate that I work for and with wonderful people and experience little or no stress at work. However, if you are having difficulties at work, you may use some of the strategies in the section on communication to get your point across. Otherwise, as you have probably figured out by now, take a trip to your local library and check out a few books on dealing with conflict resolution and stress at work. I am certain that you can find some techniques that would help you.

I should add here that you may also consider seeking professional help and counseling in dealing with your problems. There is nothing wrong in seeking help from someone with more knowledge and experience. However, keep in mind that for best

---

[31] Weiner-Davis, pp. 37–38.

results you should always try to take an active role in solving your problems by learning more about the possible solutions to them. This helps you and your therapist or counselor form a partnership and work as a team to reach the proper solution.

I hope the strategies I have discussed will be of value to you in improving the situations that cause you anger, anxiety, frustration, and resultant tension and pain. But please keep in mind that these are guidelines, and you may need to modify them to fit your individual situation or find others to deal with your particular problem. Most of all I urge you to create a balance in your life by setting goals to improve your personal, professional, family, and social life.

EPILOGUE

How can we make true progress in the management of back pain, instead of falling prey to successive fads?[1] Clinical practice should be based more firmly on the results of rigorous outcomes research, and less on seductive theories. Such research should emphasize the end results of therapy in terms of symptoms, functional status, and return to work. Finally, published research should assiduously identify possible conflicts of interest on the part of investigators. Too much research on back problems consists of case series that serve the entrepreneurial purpose of legitimizing expensive new forms of technology, rehabilitation centers, or surgical programs of uncertain effectiveness.[2]

---

[1] *Fads* here refers to ineffective treatments that become popular among physicians, such as various surgical procedures, cortisone shots, traction, transcutaneous electrical nerve stimulation, and other forms of treatment.

[2] Deyo, Richard A., "Fads in the Treatment of Low Back Pain," *The New England Journal of Medicine* 325 (1991), p. 1040. Dr. Deyo further states, "Such fads are not innocuous; they may lead to unnecessary morbidity and costs, as well as to embarrassment for professionals." In other words, some of these ineffective and baseless treatments have actually harmed patients.

When I first read this article in *The New England Journal of Medicine*, I was truly amazed. But my amazement was not because of its content, for I had discovered the same thing through months of pain and my dealings with the medical establishment. I was amazed to see profits as the reason behind the common treatments for back pain being openly admitted in such a prestigious medical journal.

Indeed, as I continue to read more about the diagnosis and treatment of back pain, I see a wide gap between what is reported in the medical journals and what is presented as facts in books available to the public.

Unfortunately, the misinformation campaign about our backs being weak and vulnerable has been so effective that not only the general public but most doctors find tension unacceptable as the cause of most back pain. Instead, most physicians insist on some structural disorder as the cause of pain.

I believe the account of my own experience with the medical community serves as clear testimony to the fact that many medical professionals are simply groping in the dark when it comes to diagnosis and treatment of back pain. Every single back patient I have come across so far was indeed suffering from TMS, and I believe Dr. Sarno's opinion, based on his decades of experience treating back patients, that most back pain is due to tension. In fact, of those I have talked to, people who accepted tension as the cause of their pain recovered quickly, but those who rejected the concept continued to suffer.

I am certain that if Tension Myositis Syndrome receives the recognition it deserves from the medical establishment, and patients are told by their doctors that tension is indeed the cause of most back pain, we will see a significant increase in the number of people who recover from chronic back pain. This will help prevent many unnecessary treatments and surgeries and save millions from pain and suffering.

Case in point: A young man I met recently had been operated on for a herniated disc four months earlier. He continued to have difficulty bending and was experiencing pain in his right leg. I briefly explained TMS to him and told him that usually the patient gets worse after the MRI shows a herniated disc. He said this was exactly what happened to him.

I asked him if he sometimes felt pain in his left leg as well, to which he replied positively. The neurosurgeon had told him the leg pain might continue for the rest of his life, because that is how back problems are. When he told the neurosurgeon that he had also been feeling pain in his hands, he was told to see a hand specialist! In the few minutes we talked, I assured him that there was nothing to worry about and suggested he read Dr. Sarno's book. And there are many more people like him who end up going from doctor to doctor and spending years in treatment while continuing to have pain or other tension-related symptoms.

But this need not be the case, as many of those who have learned about TMS have discovered. A friend of mine fell down while skiing and felt some pain in his back. One week later he woke up with sciatica in one leg; and since his brother had had a disc operation for the same condition, he became quite worried. A visit to the doctor left him with an uncertain diagnosis and a bottle of anti-inflammatory medication. I told him that as far as I could tell it was the same case as mine: TMS. I told him to take it easy, go for long walks, and try to enjoy himself for a few days. He called me two weeks later to tell me that he had been riding his bike daily, trying to relax, and no longer suffered from sciatica.

The media also contributes to our daily worries and anxieties by constantly focusing our attention on new diseases or illness, especially if one happens to be in the risk group for the reported illness or injury. Whatever part of the body is focused on, consciously or subconsciously, or is under physical stress while one is repressing anger, anxiety, and other negative emotions, will be the part of the body that begins to manifest TMS or its equivalent. A tennis player may experience tennis elbow, and a jogger may feel knee pain. Those who work with computers may experience pain in their hands. One of my friends who is a software engineer suffered from pain in his hands and back for years. He was given cortisone shots and a number of other treatments with no success. He recovered once he learned about TMS.

Today billions of dollars are spent not only on treating back-related problems but also on corrective furniture, supportive belts, and other equipment and accessories. Some companies, concerned with the staggering cost of on-the-job back "injuries," require all their employees to wear supportive belts during work hours. Add to this the millions of Americans who suffer the physical and emotional agony of chronic back pain, 2.6 million of whom are permanently disabled because of it.[3] All because the medical establishment refuses to deal with the patient as a person with a mind; what the mind experiences certainly affects the health and well being of the body.

As was demonstrated through my own experience, until the medical establishment realizes the significance of the mind/body connection, millions of people will suffer unnecessarily from this lack of vision and may become, as I did, disabled. Unless we as consumers educate ourselves and others, and are prepared to stand up for our medical rights, we cannot expect a change in this situation. I hope this book will serve as one positive step in that direction.

---

[3] Goleman, Daniel, and Joel Gurin, *Mind/Body Medicine: How to Use Your Mind for Better Health* (Yonkers, N.Y.: Consumer Report Books, 1993), p.111.

APPENDIX A

Recovery Tools

MOTIVATIONAL CHARTS

On the following page, you will find charts for "Opportunities Lost Due to Chronic Pain" and "Benefits and Pleasures of Recovering from Pain."

Write down one opportunity you missed due to chronic pain in each of the categories provided. Then, write down all the benefits and pleasures you will gain by becoming pain-free.

Post these charts near your bed or mirror as a constant reminder of why you must recover.

OPPORTUNITIES LOST DUE TO CHRONIC PAIN			
	Past	Present	Future
Personal			
Social			
Professional			
Financial			
Educational			

BENEFITS AND PLEASURES OF RECOVERING FROM PAIN	
Personal	
Social	
Professional	
Financial	
Educational	

GOALS

I have left some of the categories blank on these charts so you can enter those positions and activities that apply to your specific condition.

SHORT-TERM GOALS							
	1	2	3	4	5	6	7
GOAL							
Sit							
Stand							
Bend							

POSITIVE STATEMENT

POWER SYMBOL

REWARD

ADVANCED SHORT-TERM GOALS							
	1	2	3	4	5	6	7
GOAL							
Walk							
Climb							
Carry							

POSITIVE STATEMENT

POWER SYMBOL

REWARD

ULTIMATE LONG-TERM GOALS			
	GOAL ONE	GOAL TWO	GOAL THREE	GOAL FOUR
WEEK				
ONE				
TWO				
THREE				
FOUR				

APPENDIX B

Letters

To whom it may concern,

I am a forty-two-year-old electrical engineer with a doctorate in electrical engineering from Stanford University. I am a professor of computer engineering at University of California, Santa Cruz, and have taught at UC Berkeley Extension, Santa Clara University, and California State University, San Jose.

About three years ago, while working on the computer, I experienced severe pain in my head and neck. This was the beginning of more than eighteen months of pain in my neck and right shoulder and pain and numbness in my right arm and two fingers. I was seen by a general practitioner, two chiropractors, and eventually by a neurosurgeon at Stanford. The neurosurgeon recommended surgery based on the MRI findings. Three bulging discs were found, the worst of which was at C6-7 vertebrae. He advised me to restrict my regular sports and daily activities in order to avoid further damage to my neck.

The pain and numbness was so debilitating that I could not work on the computer for more than a few minutes at a time. I was considering major changes in my career. However, once I began using Mr. Amir's nine-step plan, I began to improve immediately. Within the first 24 hours, I was able to work on the computer an hour at a time, which was four times more than I could do one day earlier. I also increased my physical activity and one week later performed my favorite acrobatic exercise: walking on my hands!

Of course, I canceled the surgery and have not required any treatments ever since. Nowadays I keep my regular active schedule, which includes playing with my four-month-old son, teaching, and research. I hope others will also learn and benefit from Mr. Amir's recovery plan.

Dear Mr. Amir,

I want to express my deep appreciation and thanks for helping me free myself from years of pain. I suffered pain in my upper back for ten years and low back and leg pain for more than one year. My many visits to the chiropractor brought only temporary relief. As a dentist, I was worried about how this would affect my practice and my family.

However, thanks to the concepts and techniques you taught me I not only recovered completely from years of back pain, but my overall health has greatly improved as well. In fact, I have also used your methods to recover from other chronic and recurrent disorders with great success.

I recommend your nine-step recovery plan to anyone who is truly motivated to rid himself or herself from chronic pain and wants to live a healthy, active life.

Dear Fred,

It has been seven months since you helped me recover from eleven years of back, neck, and leg pain. I am writing this letter to thank you and inform others of your valuable service.

I am thirty years old and a partner in MicroBase Technologies, a computer sales and service company. Over an eleven-year period I was involved in two serious car accidents. The first time I was broadsided by a truck and taken to the hospital unconscious. I woke up later feeling pain all over and continued to have pain and muscle spasms from my left shoulder and neck down to my left leg. Therapy and medication helped, but

I continued to have pain. To make matters worse, six years later I was rear-ended on the freeway by a car traveling thirty miles faster than mine. I also suffered from pain and numbness in both forearms, wrists, and hands. My right wrist was operated on twice to relieve the pain and pressure, but I continued to have problems. As a result of all this, I was constantly in pain and was restricted in my physical activities.

When we met in February 1995 I had so much pain that I had to receive chiropractic treatment three to four times a week to relieve the pain. However, thanks to your nine-step recovery plan and caring support I was able to utilize my own strengths and abilities to recover. I am proud to report that during a recent overseas trip I was able to carry seventy-pound suitcases with complete ease and continue to enjoy a healthy and vibrant life.

Freedom from eleven years of pain feels fantastic and has been very rewarding in my personal life as well as my business—not to speak of how much time and money I have saved. I highly recommend your services to anyone seriously trying to rid themselves of chronic pain and improve their lives. It certainly worked for me.

Dear Mr. Amir,

I am writing to thank you for your help last February. As you may recall, I woke up one morning with severe pain in my left knee. The pain was so severe that I had to use a cane to walk around. I had great difficulty climbing stairs and walking. However, once I began to apply the techniques in your nine-step recovery plan I experienced rapid improvement in my condition. I was able to walk and climb stairs with much less discomfort within the first twenty-four hours and recovered completely after a few days.

As a physician, I believe your recovery plan can be of great benefit to those with chronic pain. I wish you success in your continuing efforts to help others live a pain-free life.

Dear Mr. Amir,

Thank you again for your help in my recovery from neck pain. As you know, I was involved in a head-on collision last October. Fortunately, the other car was not driving fast enough to cause life-threatening injuries. However, my car was severely damaged and I was left with pain in my neck, head, and shoulder. For three weeks I received conventional as well as chiropractic treatment, but I continued to have pain. However, the strategies in your nine-step recovery plan worked very well. I noticed an overnight improvement in my condition followed by a complete recovery.

As an electrical engineer and a test manager, I was quite concerned about the effect of chronic neck pain on my job performance. I am glad to be pain-free again and to be able to fulfill my responsibilities as a manager at work and a father of three at home. I hope many more people will benefit from your recovery plan.

Dear Mr. Amir,

I want to thank you for your help and support and recommend your program to others with back and neck pain.

I am a twenty-eight-year-old mother who suffered from chronic neck pain for five years. I also suffered from pain and numbness in my upper back, left shoulder, and arm, as well as occasional lower back and foot pain for a few months. I was diagnosed with scoliosis as the cause of my back pain. When I first learned about the strategies in your nine-step recovery plan and how effective they are, I was quite skeptical. However, I decided to try them and see if they could help me. I have to admit that within the first twelve hours there was enough improvement in my condition that I no longer needed morning massages from my husband. As I began to practice your techniques, I noticed gradual but steady improvement in pain and eventually recovered.

Dear Mr. Amir,

Thank you for your presentation on rapid recovery from chronic pain. It was great. I still cannot believe how quickly I got rid of years of pain by following your recovery plan.

For three long and painful years I suffered from pain in my heels, which began after a basketball game. I tried many different treatments, but I continued to suffer. The pain made it difficult to stand or walk for more than fifteen minutes and playing any kind of sports was out of the question. This was particularly hard on me, because I used to be very athletic and missed my active lifestyle. Although in my mid-thirties, I felt like an old man.

However, your strategies helped me recover within one day. I can stand, walk, and run without pain. I have resumed playing basketball and soccer and feel young again. I am also beginning to lose the weight I had gained due to lack of exercise. In fact, I have been so active lately that I have lost about twelve pounds since your presentation one month ago. I hope more people will have the opportunity to attend your seminars and benefit from your recovery plan.

Dear Mr. Amir,

I want to express my sincere appreciation for saving me from more than ten years of Hereditary Hemorrhagic Telangiectasia (HHT). I am one of an estimated 50,000 people with this condition in the United States. This is a hereditary disease that causes bouts of bleeding from different parts of the body. In my case I suffered from bleeding from my nose two to three times a day for the past ten years. I am a thirty-five-year-old design manager with a very responsible position at NEC Electronics. This condition was making it very difficult for me to perform at my best. In fact, once while giving a presentation I suddenly began bleeding profusely; it was quite embarrassing. Aside from the embarrassment and the inconvenience, this condition can actually be fatal; my grandfather died from excessive bleeding from his nose.

I was treated with medications and laser surgery to no avail. Nothing seemed to work until you explained to me the nine-step recovery plan. At the time I was bleeding seriously two to three times a day and experienced a serious episode right before our meeting. However, your strategies helped me improve overnight. I did not bleed at all for the following two days, experienced only a minor incident on the third day, and continued to do well. In fact, I improved so much that I was able to bend without experiencing any bleeding from my nose. Before I learned your strategies I had problem bending for more than a few seconds as this caused pressure to build up in my nose and lead to bleeding. But by the second day of your recovery plan I was able to bend completely and hold that position without bleeding.

I was also allergic to coffee, tea, and chocolate. If I had any, my nose bled. Now I drink coffee and eat as much chocolate as I want without any problems. It has been six months since my recovery and, with the exception of some minor bleeding, I have been doing great. It feels wonderful to know that I do not have to live with this condition for the rest of my life and finally can lead a normal healthy life. Thank you again and may God bless you.

Dear Fred,

It has been three years since I recovered from chronic pain in my right heel. It began as a mild discomfort and gradually became so painful that I limped when I walked. The radiology findings indicated calcium deposits in my right heel as the cause of pain, and my doctor recommended physical therapy and surgery as my treatment options.

Despite physical therapy, I continued to have pain. I had difficulty walking and standing. It seemed that surgery might be my only alternative. But when you explained your own experience with chronic pain and the steps you took to recover, I realized the possibilities for rapid recovery. I began to apply your techniques and within a few days I was not only walking, but I also began hiking, running, and eventually taking karate classes. And now after three years, I continue to do well. I wish you success with your efforts to help others.

APPENDIX C

Crucial Research

You may share the following research information with your physician or health care provider in order to determine if you need to change the course of your treatment.

Lack of Correlation Between Spinal and Disc Abnormalities and Back Pain

(arranged according to date of publication)

- Jensen, M. C., et al., "Magnetic Resonance Imaging of the Lumbar Spine in People Without Back Pain," *The New England Journal of Medicine* 331 (1994): 69–73.
- Boden, S. D., et al., "Abnormal Magnetic Resonance Scans of the Lumbar Spine in Asymptomatic Subjects," *Journal of Bone Joint Surgery* 72 (1990): 403–408.
- "Prevalence of Lumbosacral Intervertebral Disk Abnormalities on MR Images in Pregnant and Asymptomatic Nonpregnant Women," *Radiology* 170 (1989): 125-128.

- Powel, M. C., et al., "Prevalence of Lumbar Disc Degeneration Observed by Magnetic Resonance in Symptomless Women," *Lancet* 2 (1986): 1366–1377.
- Wiesel, S. W., et al., "The Incidence of Positive CAT Scans in an Asymptomatic Group of Patients," *Spine* 9 (1984): 549–551.
- Hitselberger, W. E., et al., "Abnormal Myelograms in Asymptomatic Patients," *Journal of Neurosurgery* 28 (1968): 204–206.
- McRae, D. L., "Asymptomatic Intervertebral Disc Protrusions," *acta radiol* 46 (1956): 9–27.

Ineffectiveness of Back Surgery

- U.S. Department of Health and Human Services, Agency for Health Care Policy and Research, *Understanding Acute Low Back Pain Problems*, Publication No. 95-0644 (Rockville, Md.: December 1994), p. 12. This study of 10,000 cases of back pain determined that "Surgery has been found helpful in only 1 in 100 cases of low back problems. In some people, surgery can cause more problems."

Ineffectiveness of Cortisone Shots

- Caretter, S., et al., "A Controlled Trial of Corticosteriod Injections into Facet Joints for Chronic Low Back Pain," *The New England Journal of Medicine* 325 (1991): 1001–1007. This study concluded, "Injecting methylprednisolone acetate [cortisone] into the facet joints is of little value in the treatment of patients with chronic low back pain."
- Carette S, et al., "Epidural Corticosteriod Injections for Sciatica due to Herniated Nucleus Pulposus," *The New England Journal of Medicine* 336 (1997):1634–1640. This study concluded that cortisone injections to relieve sciatica caused by a herniated disc

"offer no significant functional benefit" compared to saline solution injections.

Ineffectiveness of Back Schools

- Daltroy, Lawren H., et al., "A Controlled Trial of an Educational Program to Prevent Low Back Injuries," *The New England Journal of Medicine* 337 (1997): 332–338. Back schools are educational programs developed by physical therapists for patients with back pain. They teach good posture for sitting and standing and stretching and strengthening exercises. This study involved four thousand postal workers and compared those who had attended back schools with those who received no such training. The study found that such training did not reduce the rate of low back injury, cost per injury, time off from work per injury, rate of related injuries, or rate of repeated injury after return to work. Researchers concluded that there were "no long-term benefits associated with training."

Ineffectiveness of Treatments for Whiplash-Associated Disorders

- Spitzer, W. O., et al., "Scientific Monograph of the Quebec Task Force on Whiplash-Associated Disorders: Redefining 'Whiplash' and Its Management," *Spine* 20 (1995): 34S-39S. This comprehensive study of more than 10,000 publications on this topic revealed that the following common treatments for whiplash-associated disorders are unproven and show little or no evidence of efficacy:
  - ice
  - heat
  - laser
  - massage
  - ultrasound

- acupuncture
- cervical pillows
- muscle relaxants
- spray and stretch
- psychosocial intervention
- postural alignment training
- epidural or intrathecal injections
- transcutaneous electrical stimulation

Ineffectiveness of Surgery for Carpal Tunnel Syndrome

- Surgery for carpal tunnel syndrome has also been found ineffective: "Correcting carpal tunnel syndrome is one of the most common operations performed today. The only problem is, it often doesn't work," concluded researchers at the Washington University School of Medicine in St. Louis ("Surgery Often Useless for Carpal Tunnel Pain," *San Jose Mercury News*, February 22, 1995).

The above findings are applicable to many chronic pain conditions. For example, if you suffer from chronic or recurrent neck pain, the treatments that are ineffective for whiplash or back pain are obviously ineffective for neck pain. Since back surgery fails 99 percent of the time to help patients, it is reasonable to conclude that it does not have a good success rate in helping patients with neck pain.

You, as a patient and a consumer, must exercise good judgment in utilizing the above information and form a partnership with your health care provider in order to find the appropriate course of treatment for your condition.

BIBLIOGRAPHY

BACK PAIN

Calliet, Rene, M.D., *Low Back Pain Syndrome*, 4th ed. (Philadelphia: F. A. Davis Co., 1988).

Editors of Lanier Publishing, *The Back Almanac* (Berkeley, Calif.: Ten Speed Press, 1992).

Klien, Arthur, and Dava Sobel, *Backache Relief* (New York: Penguin Books, 1985).

Sarno, John, M.D., *Healing Back Pain* (New York: Warner Books, 1991).

Sarno, John, M.D., *Mind over Back Pain* (New York: William Morrow & Co, 1984).

Sarno, John E., *The Mindbody Prescription: Healing the Body, Healing the Pain* (New York: Warner Books, 1998).

Zimmerman, Julie, P.T., *Chronic Back Pain: Moving On.* (Brunswick, Maine: Biddle Publishing Co., 1991).

Zimmerman, Julie, P.T., *The Diagnosis and Misdiagnosis of Back Pain* (Brunswick, Maine: Biddle Publishing Co., 1991).

MIND AND BODY

Benson, Herbert, M.D., *Your Maximum Mind* (New York: Times Books, 1989).

Benson, Herbert, *Timeless Healing: The Power and Biology of Belief* (New York: Scribner, 1996).

Cousins, Norman, *Head First: The Biology of Hope* (New York: Dutton, 1989).

Epstein, Gerald, M.D., *Healing Visualization: Creating Health Through Imagery* (New York: Bantam Books, 1989).

Faelton, Sharon, and David Diamond, *Tension Turnaround* (Emmaus, Pa: Rodale Press, 1990).

Fiore, Neil, and Lloyd Glauberman. *Turn Off Tension* (Los Angeles: Audio Renaissance Tapes, 1990).

Goleman, Daniel, and Joel Gurin, *Mind/Body Medicine: How to Use Your Mind for Better Health* (Yonkers, N.Y.: Consumer Report Books, 1993).

Goleman, Daniel, *Emotional Intelligence* (New York: Bantam Books, 1995).

Moyers, Bill, *Healing and the Mind* (New York: Doubleday, 1993).

Ornstein, Robert, Ph.D., and David Sobel, M.D., *The Healing Brain* (New York: Simon & Shuster, 1987).

Padus, Emrika, *The Complete Guide to Your Emotions and Your Health* (Emmaus, Pa: Rodale Press, 1992).

Pellteier, Kenneth. M.D., *Sound Mind, Sound Body* (New York: Simon & Shuster, 1994).

Rossman, Martin, M.D., *Healing Yourself: A Step-by-Step Program to Better Health by Imagery.* (New York: Walker, 1987).

Samuels, Michael, M.D., and Samuels, Nancy, *Healing with the Mind's Eye* (New York: Summit Books, 1990).

Wells, Valerie, *The Joy of Visualization: 75 Creative Ways to Enhance Your Life* (San Francisco: Chronicle Books, 1990).

WELLNESS

Bates, William, M.D., *Better Eyesight Without Glasses* (New York: Henry Holt and Co., 1940, 1971).

Benson, Herbert, M.D. and Eileen Stuart, R.N., *The Wellness Book.* (New York: Fireside Books, 1993).

Carper, Jeane, *Food: Your Miracle Medicine* (New York: HarperCollins, 1993).

Carper, Jean, *Miracle Cures: Dramatic New Scientific Discoveries Revealing the Healing Powers of Herbs, Vitamins, and Other Natural Remedies* (New York: HarperCollins Publishers, 1997).

Editors of Boardroom Classics, *Healing Unlimited* (New York: Boardroom Reports, 1994).

Huxley, Aldous, *The Art of Seeing* (Berkeley, Calif.: Creative Arts Publishing, 1982).

Michuad, Ellen, and Alice Feinstein *Prevention Magazine's 30-Day Immune Power Program* (Emmaus, Pa: Rodale Press, 1992).

Ornstein, Robert, Ph.D., and David Sobel, M.D., *Healthy Pleasures* (Reading, Mass: Addison-Wesley, 1989).

Travis, John, M.D., and Regina S. Ryan, *Wellness: Small Changes You Can Use to Make a Big Difference* (Berkeley, Calif.: Ten Speed Press, 1988).

Salaman, Maureen, *Foods That Heal* (Menlo Park, Calif.: Statford Publishing, 1989).

Weil, Andrew, M.D., *Natural Health, Natural Medicine: A Comprehensive Manual for Wellness and Self-Care* (Boston: Houghton Mifflin, 1990).

Weil, Andrew, M.D., *Spontaneous Healing: How to Discover and Enhance Your Body's Natural Ability to Maintain and Heal Itself* (New York: Knopf, 1995).

Weil, Andrew, *Eight Weeks to Optimum Health* (New York: Alfred A. Knopf, 1997).

HEALTH AND FITNESS

Bailey, Covert, *The New Fit or Fat* (Boston: Houghton Mifflin Co., 1991).

Bailey, Covert, *Smart Exercise* (Boston: Houghton Mifflin Co., 1994).

Cooper, Robert, Ph.D., *Health and Fitness Excellence: The Scientific Action Plan* (Boston: Houghton Mifflin Co., 1989).

Evans, William J., M.D., *Biomarkers: The 10 Keys to Prolonging Vitality* (New York: Fireside Books, 1991).

Pearl, Bill, *Getting Stronger: Weight Training for Men and Women* (Bolinas, Calif.: Shelter Publishing Co., 1986).

MEDICINE

Arnot, Robert, M.D., *The Best Medicine: How to Choose the Top Doctors, and the Top Hospitals, and the Top Treatments* (Reading, Mass.: Addison-Wesley, 1992).

Editors of Prevention Magazine, *The Doctors Book of Home Remedies* (Emmaus, Pa.: Rodale Press, 1990).

Inlander, Charles, *Medicine on Trial: The Appalling Story of Ineptitude, Malfeasance, Neglect, and Arrogance* (New York: Prentice Hall Press, 1988).

Inlander, Charles, *Take This Book to The Hospital With You* (Emmaus, Pa.: Rodale Press, 1985).

Inlander, Charles, *Your Medical Rights* (Boston: Little Brown, 1990).

Inlander, Charles B., *Good Operations–Bad Operations: The People's Medical Society's Guide to Surgery* (New York: Viking, 1993).

Isaacs, Stephen, J.D., *The Consumer's Legal Guide to Today's Health Care: Your Medical Rights and How to Assert Them* (Boston: Houghton Mifflin Co., 1992).

Kemp, C.H., et al., *Current Pediatric Diagnosis and Treatment.* 9th ed. (Norwalk, Conn: Appleton and Lange, 1987).

Ornish, Dean, M.D., *Dr. Ornish's Program for Reversing Heart Disease* (New York: Random House, 1990).

Payer, Lynn, *Disease-Mongers: How Doctors, Drug Companies, and Insurers Are Making You Feel Sick* (New York: John Wiley & Sons, 1992).

Peikin, Steven, M.D., *Gastrointestinal Health* (New York: HarperCollins Publishers, 1991).

Pell, Arthur, Ph.D., *Diagnosing Your Doctor: A Straightforward Guide to Asking the Right Questions and Getting the Health*

Care You Deserve (Minneapolis: Chromined Publishing, 1991).

Walzer, Richard, M.D., *Healthy Skin: A Guide For Life Long Skin Care* (Mt. Vermont, NY: Consumer Union, 1989).

GENERAL INTEREST

Atkinson, Rita, et al., *Introduction to Psychology* (New York: Harcourt Brace Jovanovich Publishers, 1990).

Coloroso, Barbara, *Kids Are Worth It! Giving Your Child the Gift of Inner Discipline* (New York: William Morrow and Co. 1994).

Covey, Stephen R., et al., *First Things First* (New York: Simon & Shuster. 1994).

Dossey, Larry, M.D., *Healing Words: The Power of Prayer and the Practice of Medicine* (San Francisco: Harper San Francisco, 1993).

Editors and Experts of *Bottom Line Personal, The Book of Inside Information* (New York: Boardroom Reports, 1992).

Gray, John, Ph.D.. *Men Are from Mars, Women Are from Venus* (New York: Harper Collins Publishers, 1992).

Gray, John, *Mars and Venus Together Forever: Relationship Skills for Lasting Love Last* (New York: HarperPerennial, 1996).

Helmstetter, Shad, Ph.D., *The Self-Talk Solution* (New York: William Morrow and Co., 1987).

Helmstetter, Shad, Ph.D., *What To Say When You Talk To Yourself* (New York: Pocket Books, 1982).

Kabat-Zinn, Jon, Ph.D., *Full Catastrophe Living: Using the Wisdom of Your Body and Mind to Face Stress, Pain, and Illness* (New York: Delacorte Press, 1990).

Johnson, Spencer, M.D., *The One Minute Father* (New York: William Morrow and Co. 1983).

Johnson, Spencer, M.D., *The One Minute Mother* (New York: William Morrow and Co. 1983).

Mayson, L. John, *Guide to Stress Reduction* (Berkeley, Calif.: Celestial Arts, 1985).

Ornish, Dean, *Love and Survival: The Scientific Basis for the Healing Power of Intimacy* (New York: HarperCollins, 1998).

Pryor, Karen, *Don't Shoot the Dog* (New York: Simon and Shuster, 1984).

Robbins, Anthony, *Awaken The Giant Within* (New York: Summit Books, 1991).

Robbins Anthony, *Unlimited Power* (New York: Ballantine Books, 1986).

Rosenbaum, Edward, M.D., *A Taste of My Own Medicine* (New York: Random House. 1988).

Tannen, Barbara, *You Just Don't Understand: Women and Men in Conversation* (New York: William Morrow and Co. 1990).

Weiner-Davis, Michele, *Divorce Busting: A Revolutionary and Rapid Program for Staying Together* (New York: Summit Books, 1992).

Wurtman, Judith J., Ph.D., *Managing Your Mind and Mood Through Food* (New York: HarperCollins, 1987).

Wurtman, Judith, *The Serotonin Solution* (New York: Fawcett Columbine, 1997).

GLOSSARY

Acupressure. Treatment approach using deep thumb or finger pressure on acupuncture points.

Acupuncture. Insertion of needles into certain parts of the body to decrease pain.

Arthritis. Refers to inflammation of joints.

Autonomic nervous system. Portion of the nervous system that regulates breathing, heart rate, blood pressure, glands, and other bodily functions.

Behavior modification. This is a therapeutic approach in which a systematic attempt is made to change learned behavior patterns by utilizing the principles of conditioning.

Body mechanics. The posture of the body in motion.

CAT scan. Abbreviation for computerized axial tomography. Specialized X-ray technique that reveals three planes of bones, joints, and organs. Reveals soft tissues as well as bones.

Chronic back pain. A back pain lasting longer than three months.

Conditioning. This happens when a previously neutral stimulus becomes capable of eliciting a learned response. Russian physiologist Ivan Pavlov rang a bell (stimulus) every time he fed the dogs. Soon the dogs would salivate (learned response) whenever they heard a bell ring, even though there was no food present. In back pain many previously neutral actions and positions such as bending and sitting have become a conditioned response and cause pain. The pain began due to tension but now has become a learned response.

Chondromalacia patella. Refers to the roughening of the underside of the patella (knee cap).

Cortisone. A hormone with anti-inflammatory properties injected into muscles, joints, or discs suspected of causing pain.

Defense mechanisms. The strategy used by the mind to ward off or to reduce anxiety. These consist of adjustments made subconsciously (unconsciously) either through action or avoidance of action, to keep from facing unacceptable personal motives or unpleasant, harsh realities of unacceptable circumstances, such as sudden death of a loved one. Denial and regression are two examples of defense mechanisms.

Degenerated disc. A thinning of the disc that is due to aging and use, especially in the lower back and neck area. This is a common and normal condition and not responsible for back or neck pain.

Denial. When a person faces an unacceptable, unpleasant circumstance, such as the sudden death of a loved one, he or she might deny this really happened. This denial serves as a defense mechanism to protect the person from facing the harsh reality.

Desensitization. This is a form of psychotherapy in which a patient learns to eliminate unwanted emotional responses to certain stimuli (words, objects, situations, etc.). This is accomplished through a process of repeated exposure to these stimuli in life or in one's imagination.

Disc. A water-containing gelatinous mass surrounded by fibers, between two spinal vertebrae; it acts to cushion the vertebrae and permit spinal flexibility.

Electromyography (EMG). Diagnostic test in which needle electrodes inserted into muscle tissue relay electrical impulses from the muscle in order to identify nervous system diseases.

Ergonomics. Adaptation of the workplace and equipment to accommodate an injured worker or to prevent injuries.

Gastritis. Inflammation of the stomach lining.

Herniated disc. Means the disc material has been forced out of its normal position between two adjacent vertebrae and has entered into the spinal column.

Lumbar spine. Refers to the lower back, the five vertebrae below the thoracic spine and the sacrum.

Magnetic resonance imaging (MRI). A non-invasive diagnostic test in which magnetic waves are used to image soft tissues.

Orthopedic surgeon. A medical doctor specializing in musculoskeletal surgery.

Osteoarthritis. Refers to the localized degenerative changes in joints.

Physiatrist. A medical doctor specializing in physical medicine and non-surgical rehabilitation.

Piriformis. A muscle in the buttock area that helps in rotation of the hip through or under which the sciatic nerve passes.

Positive reinforcement. This is a positive stimulus (encouragement, reward, etc.) used in conditioning to increase the occurrence of a response.

Regression. This concept suggests that when faced with conflict, stress, and particular frustration, a person may return to an earlier stage of life in which the person was secure, and in so doing avoid facing the present unpleasant, stressful situation.

Rheumatologist. A medical doctor specializing in diseases of the joints such as arthritis.

Ruptured disc. *See* Herniated disc.

Sciatica. Refers to the pain, irritation, and other discomforting sensations associated with the sciatic nerve, which runs down the back of the leg.

Sciatic nerve. Large nerve formed by numerous nerves that become united into one major nerve within the pelvis and runs down the back of the thigh and innervates the posterior thigh, lower leg, and foot.

Scoliosis. Lateral curvature of the spine, not a cause of back pain.

Shiatsu. This is a massage therapy that uses acupressure to relieve pain.

Subconscious mind. This is the level of mental activity assumed to exist just below the threshold of consciousness.

Tendonitis. Inflammation of the tendon.

Tension Myositis Syndrome (TMS). Refers to an extremely painful, yet harmless, condition in which muscles, nerves, tendons, and ligaments are deprived of oxygen due to repressed anger, fear, anxiety, and tension.

Type A personality. Refers to a type of personality dominated by aggressive, impatient, and tense behavior.

Zantac. An ulcer medication that reduces stomach acid.

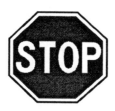

Help Someone in Pain

Share the empowering concepts and effective strategies presented in *Rapid Recovery from Back and Neck Pain* with loved ones, friends, and coworkers. Help them avoid unnecessary tests and procedures and ineffective treatments. Help them get on the road to wellness and a pain-free, productive life.

Give the gift of knowledge and good health by ordering *Rapid Recovery from Back and Neck Pain* for just $14.97 per copy, plus 10% for shipping and handling* (minimum $3.50). California residents, please add 8.25% sales tax. For international orders shipping charges are $6 for Canada, $10 for Europe and Australia, $12.00 for Asia and Africa for one book and $2 for additional books.

Mail your check or money order to
Health Advisory Group, LLC
2464 El Camino Real, PMB 157
Santa Clara, CA 95051

Please include your name, complete shipping address, and daytime telephone number or e-mail address.

If you would like to order by credit card, please logon to www.rapidrecovery.net.

Thank you for helping someone get rid of the pain.
Allow up to two weeks for delivery.